A Summary of the December 2009
Forum on the Future of Nursing

CARE IN THE COMMUNITY

Committee on the Robert Wood Johnson
Foundation Initiative on the Future of Nursing,
at the Institute of Medicine

INSTITUTE OF MEDICINE
OF THE NATIONAL ACADEMIES

THE NATIONAL ACADEMIES PRESS
Washington, D.C.
www.nap.edu

THE NATIONAL ACADEMIES PRESS • 500 Fifth Street, N.W. • Washington, DC 20001

NOTICE: The project that is the subject of this report was approved by the Governing Board of the National Research Council, whose members are drawn from the councils of the National Academy of Sciences, the National Academy of Engineering, and the Institute of Medicine. The members of the committee responsible for the report were chosen for their special competences and with regard for appropriate balance.

Support for this project was provided by the Robert Wood Johnson Foundation. Any opinions, findings, conclusions, or recommendations expressed in this publication are those of the author(s) and do not necessarily reflect the views of the organizations or agencies that provided support for the project.

International Standard Book Number-13: 978-0-309-15279-2
International Standard Book Number-10: 0-309-15279-8

Additional copies of this report are available from the National Academies Press, 500 Fifth Street, N.W., Lockbox 285, Washington, DC 20055; (800) 624-6242 or (202) 334-3313 (in the Washington metropolitan area); Internet, http://www.nap.edu.

For more information about the Institute of Medicine, visit the IOM home page at: **www.iom.edu.**

Printed in the United States of America

Cover credit: Top photo © 2010 Gregory Benson. Bottom photos reprinted with permission from USeventPhotos.com.

Suggested citation: IOM (Institute of Medicine). 2010. *A summary of the December 2009 forum on the future of nursing: Care in the community.* Washington, DC: The National Academies Press.

"Knowing is not enough; we must apply.
Willing is not enough; we must do."
—Goethe

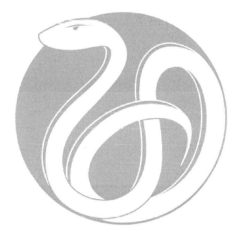

INSTITUTE OF MEDICINE
OF THE NATIONAL ACADEMIES

Advising the Nation. Improving Health.

THE NATIONAL ACADEMIES
Advisers to the Nation on Science, Engineering, and Medicine

The **National Academy of Sciences** is a private, nonprofit, self-perpetuating society of distinguished scholars engaged in scientific and engineering research, dedicated to the furtherance of science and technology and to their use for the general welfare. Upon the authority of the charter granted to it by the Congress in 1863, the Academy has a mandate that requires it to advise the federal government on scientific and technical matters. Dr. Ralph J. Cicerone is president of the National Academy of Sciences.

The **National Academy of Engineering** was established in 1964, under the charter of the National Academy of Sciences, as a parallel organization of outstanding engineers. It is autonomous in its administration and in the selection of its members, sharing with the National Academy of Sciences the responsibility for advising the federal government. The National Academy of Engineering also sponsors engineering programs aimed at meeting national needs, encourages education and research, and recognizes the superior achievements of engineers. Dr. Charles M. Vest is president of the National Academy of Engineering.

The **Institute of Medicine** was established in 1970 by the National Academy of Sciences to secure the services of eminent members of appropriate professions in the examination of policy matters pertaining to the health of the public. The Institute acts under the responsibility given to the National Academy of Sciences by its congressional charter to be an adviser to the federal government and, upon its own initiative, to identify issues of medical care, research, and education. Dr. Harvey V. Fineberg is president of the Institute of Medicine.

The **National Research Council** was organized by the National Academy of Sciences in 1916 to associate the broad community of science and technology with the Academy's purposes of furthering knowledge and advising the federal government. Functioning in accordance with general policies determined by the Academy, the Council has become the principal operating agency of both the National Academy of Sciences and the National Academy of Engineering in providing services to the government, the public, and the scientific and engineering communities. The Council is administered jointly by both Academies and the Institute of Medicine. Dr. Ralph J. Cicerone and Dr. Charles M. Vest are chair and vice chair, respectively, of the National Research Council.

www.national-academies.org

COMMITTEE ON THE ROBERT WOOD JOHNSON FOUNDATION INITIATIVE ON THE FUTURE OF NURSING, AT THE INSTITUTE OF MEDICINE

DONNA E. SHALALA (*Chair*), University of Miami, Coral Gables, FL
LINDA BURNES BOLTON (*Vice Chair*), Cedars-Sinai Health System and Research Institute, Los Angeles, CA
MICHAEL BLEICH, Oregon Health & Science University School of Nursing, Portland
TROYEN (TROY) A. BRENNAN, CVS Caremark, Woonsocket, RI
ROBERT E. CAMPBELL, Johnson & Johnson (*retired*), New Brunswick, NJ
LEAH DEVLIN, University of North Carolina at Chapel Hill, School of Public Health
CATHERINE DOWER, University of California–San Francisco
ROSA GONZALEZ-GUARDA, University of Miami, Coral Gables, FL
DAVID C. GOODMAN, Dartmouth Medical School, Hanover, NH
JENNIE CHIN HANSEN, AARP, Washington, DC
C. MARTIN HARRIS, Cleveland Clinic, Cleveland, OH
ANJLI AURORA HINMAN, Intown Midwifery, Atlanta, GA
WILLIAM D. NOVELLI, Georgetown University, Washington, DC
LIANA ORSOLINI-HAIN, City College of San Francisco, CA
YOLANDA PARTIDA, University of California–San Francisco, Fresno
ROBERT D. REISCHAUER, Urban Institute, Washington, DC
JOHN W. ROWE, Columbia University, New York
BRUCE C. VLADECK, Nexera Consulting, New York

Study Staff
JUDITH A. SALERNO, Executive Officer
SUSAN HASSMILLER, Director, Robert Wood Johnson Foundation Initiative on the Future of Nursing, at the Institute of Medicine
ADRIENNE STITH BUTLER, Senior Program Officer
ANDREA M. SCHULTZ, Associate Program Officer
KATHARINE BOTHNER, Research Associate
THELMA L. COX, Administrative Assistant
TONIA E. DICKERSON, Senior Program Assistant
GINA IVEY, Communications Director, Robert Wood Johnson Foundation Initiative on the Future of Nursing, at the Institute of Medicine

LORI MELICHAR, Research Director, Robert Wood Johnson Foundation Initiative on the Future of Nursing, at the Institute of Medicine
JULIE FAIRMAN, Nurse Scholar-in-Residence

Consultants
PAUL LIGHT, New York University
STEVE OLSON, Technical Writer
JOSEF REUM, George Washington University, Washington, DC

Reviewers

This report has been reviewed in draft form by individuals chosen for their diverse perspectives and technical expertise, in accordance with procedures approved by the National Research Council's Report Review Committee. The purpose of this independent review is to provide candid and critical comments that will assist the institution in making its published report as sound as possible and to ensure that the report meets institutional standards for objectivity, evidence, and responsiveness to the study charge. The review comments and draft manuscript remain confidential to protect the integrity of the process. We wish to thank the following individuals for their review of this report:

Patricia Gerrity, Eleventh Street Family Health Services of Drexel University

Tine Hansen-Turton, National Nursing Centers Consortium and Public Health Management Corporation

Charlene A. Harrington, University of California, San Francisco

Mel Worth, Emeritus Scholar, Institute of Medicine

Although the reviewers listed above have provided many constructive comments and suggestions, they were not asked to endorse the final draft of the report before its release. The review of this report was overseen by **Ada Sue Hinshaw,** Graduate School of Nursing, Uniformed Services University of the Health Sciences. Appointed by the National Research Council and the Institute of Medicine, she was responsible for making certain that an independent examination of this report was carried out in accordance with institutional procedures and that all review comments were carefully considered. Responsibility for the final content of this report rests entirely with the authors and the institution.

Preface

In 2009 the Initiative on the Future of Nursing, a collaborative effort between the Robert Wood Johnson Foundation (RWJF) and the Institute of Medicine (IOM), undertook a major study on the future of nursing during a critical period in the history of the U.S. health care system. The health care reform debate in Congress and throughout the nation revealed many questions and unknowns. Yet one theme to emerge was the necessary re-examination and re-imagination of the role of nurses to take on challenges facing the profession and to help fulfill the promise of a re-formed health care system—improving health. The charge of the RWJF Initiative on the Future of Nursing, at the IOM, is to recommend changes in public and institutional policies at the federal, state, and local levels in order to provide a blueprint for action for the future of nursing.

On December 3, 2009, the initiative held its second public forum at the Community College of Philadelphia. The forums were designed to inform the committee about the critical and varied roles of nurses across settings. With opening remarks by Governor Edward Rendell on health care reform efforts in Pennsylvania, this forum examined the future of nursing in the community, focusing on community health, public health, primary care, and long-term care. This forum was especially important to the committee since care is increasingly being provided in non-acute settings and is more focused on disease prevention, health promotion, and chronic illness management. While well over half of all nurses practice in acute care settings, nurses in community settings are vital to ensuring access to quality care.

More than 200 forum attendees—and an even larger audience watching the live webcast—heard a series of presentations from leaders in the field, including testimony from 15 individuals representing a variety of organizations and personal views. Prior to the forum, several members of the IOM committee visited a number of community-based health centers across Philadelphia. Concluding the day's events, 30 RWJF fellows and scholars reviewed their observations at the forum and site visits to develop a set of relevant recommendations for the committee's consideration. It was an informative and often eye-opening day for the committee members and RWJF fellows and scholars who attended the events.

The forum presenters described a segment of best practices in the community that shed light on what is currently available and what will be required to meet the changing health needs of the diverse populations of this country. As a result of this forum, the committee was given an opportunity to consider how changing health needs in the community will affect the future of the nursing profession in terms of the way care is delivered, the setting in which care is provided, and the education requirements for the necessary skills and competencies to provide quality care.

Many important messages emerged from the forum, including:

- Budgets for public health and community health programs are being cut at a time when these programs are needed most to care for aging populations and when greater emphasis is being placed on prevention, wellness, chronic disease management, and moving care into the community.
- Nursing in the community occurs through partnerships with many other individuals and organizations, and nurses need to take a leadership role in establishing these vital partnerships. Fostering this type of collaboration could improve the continuum of care between acute and community care settings.
- Technology has the potential to transform the lives of nurses providing care in the community, as well as their patients, just as it is transforming commerce, education, communications, and entertainment for the public.
- Varying scopes of practice across states have, in some cases, prevented nurses from providing care to the fullest extent possible at the community level.
- Nurse-managed health clinics offer opportunities to expand access; provide quality, evidence-based care; and improve outcomes for individuals who may not otherwise receive needed care. These clinics also provide the necessary support to engage individuals in wellness and prevention activities.

- Nursing students need to have greater exposure to principles of community care, leadership, and care provision through changes in nursing school curricula and increased opportunities to gain experience in community care settings.
- The delivery of quality nursing care has the potential to provide value across community settings and can be achieved though effective leadership, policy, and accountability.

At one point during the forum, the moderator, Dr. Joseph Reum, interim dean of the School of Public Health and Health Services at the George Washington University, asked members of the audience to consider how nursing would be different if all of the barriers to change suddenly disappeared. The responses were fascinating. One respondent said that she would have access to a nurse whenever she needed one. Nurses would be members of interdisciplinary teams that would care for individuals from birth to death, said another attendee. Nurses would provide care in all settings, was a third response, from hospitals to home and everywhere in between—schools, churches, community centers, health departments, long-term care facilities. Nurses would have instant access to electronic medical records, said a fourth person, so that they always have the information they need to provide the best possible care.

The committee is developing a set of recommendations that will lead to bold changes in nursing and will help ensure the health of Americans. The forum in Philadelphia gave us not only ideas but also hope that such change is possible. As Mary Selecky, the secretary of the Washington State Department of Health, said in her keynote address, "It is time to seize the moment, to step up to the challenge, and to create the future that should be."

Donna E. Shalala
Committee Chair

Jennie Chin Hansen
Committee Member and
Forum Planning Group Chair

Acknowledgments

The Robert Wood Johnson Foundation (RWJF) Initiative on the Future of Nursing, at the Institute of Medicine (IOM), wishes to thank the numerous individuals and organizations that contributed to the success of the Forum on the Future of Nursing: Care in the Community. The forum was graciously hosted by the Community College of Philadelphia; its staff, particularly Elaine Tagliareni, Monique Westcott, and Joe McFadden, provided invaluable support throughout the planning and execution of the forum.

The initiative would like to thank Josef Reum for his facilitation skills, as well as the speakers, panelists, and all who provided testimony throughout the forum; the insight and experience that was shared throughout the day greatly contributed to the deliberations of the committee. The initiative would also like to recognize the alumni from various RWJF fellow and scholar programs who participated in the forum. These individuals gathered to reflect on the day's discussions and offered the committee several thoughtful and innovative ideas to consider for the future of nursing in community care settings.

While in Philadelphia, the initiative visited several community health centers and would like to express gratitude to the following individuals for warmly welcoming us into their facilities and providing us with on-the-ground perspectives of nursing care across community settings: Joan Bland at the Philadelphia Department of Health, Community Health Center #3; Kent Bream at the Sayre School-Based Health Clinic; Patricia Gerrity at the 11th Street Family Health Services of Drexel University; Eileen Sullivan Marx at the LIFE Program; Nancy Rothman at the Health Connection; and Donna Torisi and Lorraine Thomas at the Health Annex.

The forum could not have happened without the expertise and leadership of the committee planning group. The planning group was chaired by Jennie Chin Hansen and included Michael Bleich, Troy Brennan, Leah Devlin, Anjli Aurora Hinman, Yolanda Partida, John Rowe, and Donna E. Shalala.

For their steadfast and creative work throughout the course of the forum, we would like to recognize the Initiative staff members, led by Susan Hassmiller and Adrienne Stith Butler, with guidance and oversight from Judith Salerno. The following individuals were involved in planning the forum, day-of support, and the production of this summary: Katharine Bothner, Thelma Cox, Julie Dashiell, Tonia Dickerson, Gina Ivey, Lori Melichar, Abbey Meltzer, and Andrea Schultz. The forum was webcast by ON24 and transcribed by Joy Biletz. The Initiative is grateful to Steve Olson for his editorial and writing assistance, to Florence Poillon for copyediting the summary, and to Dan Banks for designing the cover. We would also like to recognize the contributions of the following staff and consultants to this activity: Clyde Behney, Christie Bell, Julie Fairman, Christine Gorman, Amy Levey, Paul Light, Tamara Parr, Sharon Reis, Christine Stencel, Vilija Teel, Lauren Tobias, Jackie Turner, Gary Walker, and Jordan Wyndelts.

Finally, the Initiative would like to express its appreciation to the RWJF, whose generous financial support, and mission to improve the health and health care of all Americans, made the forum possible.

Contents

1 INTRODUCTION   **1**
Site Visits, 2
Forum Welcome: A Laboratory for Health Care Reform, 3

2 PUBLIC POLICY AND PUBLIC HEALTH NURSING   **7**
Challenges Facing Public Health Nurses, 8
Public Policy Implications, 10
Responses to Questions, 12

3 COMMUNITY AND PUBLIC HEALTH   **15**
Nursing in the Community, 15
The Future of Nurses in Community Care, 19
Responses to Questions, 22

4 PRIMARY CARE   **25**
Nurse Practitioners as Leaders in Primary Care, 25
The Indian Health Service: A Rural Health Care Service, 29
Responses to Questions, 33

**5 CHRONIC AND LONG-TERM SERVICES
AND SUPPORTS**   **35**
Nurses' Roles in Meeting Long-Term Health Care Needs, 35
Evercare Models of Nursing, 37
Responses to Questions, 39

6 TESTIMONY   **41**

APPENDIXES

A   References   **59**
B   Agenda   **63**
C   Speaker Biosketches   **65**

1

Introduction

On December 3, 2009, the Initiative on the Future of Nursing, a collaborative effort between the Robert Wood Johnson Foundation (RWJF) and the Institute of Medicine (IOM), held a forum at the Community College of Philadelphia to examine the challenges facing the nursing profession with regard to care in the community, including aspects of community health, public health, primary care, and long-term care. The forum was the second of three held to gather information and discuss ideas related to the future of nursing. The first forum held October 19, 2009, at Cedars-Sinai Medical Center in Los Angeles, focused on the future of nursing in acute care. The third forum, on February 22, 2010, in Houston, examined the future of nursing education.

The forums have been part of an intensive information-gathering effort by an IOM committee that is the cornerstone of the Initiative on the Future of Nursing. The committee will use the information collected at these forums, at its two technical workshops, from data provided by the RWJF Nursing Research Network, and from a number of commissioned papers to inform the development of its findings, conclusions, and recommendations. The committee's final recommendations will be presented in a report on the capacity of the nursing workforce to meet the demands of a reformed health care system.

Each of the three forums was planned with the guidance of a small group of committee members; the planning group for this forum was led by Ms. Jennie Chin Hansen. The half-day forums were not meant to be an exhaustive examination of all settings in which nurses practice or of the complexity of the nursing profession as a whole. Given the limited amount of time for each of the three forums, a comprehensive review of all facets and all players of each of the main forum themes was not possible. Rather, the forums were meant to inform the committee on important topics within the nursing profession and to highlight some of the key challenges, barriers, opportunities, and innovations that nurses face while working in an evolving health care system. Many of the critical challenges, barriers, opportunities, and innovations discussed at the forums overlap across settings and throughout the nursing profession and also are applicable to other providers and individuals who work with nurses.

This summary of the forum on care in the community describes the main points made by speakers in their presentations and during the discussion and question-and-answer periods that followed, as well as points made by forum participants who offered testimony. A complete agenda of the forum can be found in Appendix B, and biosketches of the speakers can be found in Appendix C. The remaining sections of this chapter describe two activities that occurred in conjunction with the forum and also present the welcoming remarks of Pennsylvania Governor Edward Rendell. Chapter 2 summarizes the talk of keynote speaker Mary C. Selecky. Chapters 3, 4, and 5 describe the remarks and answers to questions at sessions focused on community and public health, primary care, and chronic and long-term care, respectively. Chapter 6 summarizes the oral testimony presented by 15 forum attendees, along with remarks made by forum participants during an open-microphone session at the end of the forum.

Comments made at the forum should not be interpreted as positions of the committee, RWJF, IOM, or the Community College of Pennsylvania. Committee members' questions and comments do not necessarily reflect their personal views or the conclusions that will be in the committee's report. However, the questions and comments were designed to elicit information and perspectives that can guide the committee's deliberations.

SITE VISITS

In the morning before the forum began, the committee members participated in a series of site visits throughout the city of Philadelphia to community and public health centers, some of which were nurse-led and managed. During the site visits they had the opportunity to talk with nurses, administrators, other health care providers, and patients about some of the challenges and innovative strategies that nurses are using in these settings to provide quality care in the community and expand access. Observations made during these site visits are not part of this summary of the forum, but the site visits informed at least some of the questions directed to speakers by committee members at the event. The six sites visited by committee members were the Living Independently for Elders (LIFE) program at the University of Pennsylvania School of Nursing, the Sayre High School School-Based Health Clinic, Community Health Center #3 of the Philadelphia Department of Health, Health Annex, Health Connections, and the 11th Street Family Health Services of Drexel University.

Robert Wood Johnson Foundation Solutions Session

After the forum, a select group of RWJF scholars and fellows hosted by RWJF met to discuss what they saw on the site visits and heard at the forum in the context of their own expertise, knowledge, and judgment. This session was independent of the IOM committee and the forum on the future of nursing. The goal of the session was to provide an opportunity for the fellows and scholars to consider solutions and the most promising future roles for nurses in public health, community health, primary care, and long-term care.

The solutions offered by the fellows and scholars are not described in this summary of the forum. However, summaries of their solutions were provided to the committee for its review and consideration at the committee's subsequent meeting in January 2010.

FORUM WELCOME:
A LABORATORY FOR HEALTH CARE REFORM

The states have historically been laboratories for public policy, said Pennsylvania Governor Edward Rendell in his opening remarks at the forum. If new ideas are successful in one state, other states and the federal government may adopt those ideas. States, including Pennsylvania, have played a particularly important role in experimenting with innovative health care reform strategies. When Rendell became governor of Pennsylvania in 2003, "there was no chance for comprehensive national health care reform and no guarantee that it would happen in the next decade." The state stepped into the breech by launching a comprehensive reform program called Prescription for Pennsylvania, which Rendell noted has become a model for the federal government in implementing national health care reform.

The mission of Prescription for Pennsylvania, said Rendell, "was to ensure that every resident of Pennsylvania had access to quality, affordable health care." That meant dealing with issues of both access and cost, and one of the first things the state realized is that nurses could help resolve both of those problems. The addition of a nurse practitioner to a medical practice can double the number of patients seen while maintaining the same level of quality and lowering costs (AANP, 2007). To take advantage of these savings and expand access to care, Pennsylvania broadened the scope of practice for nurse practitioners, allowing an expansion of the number of clinics run by nurses in a variety of settings, including retail locations. Since Prescription for Pennsylvania moved forward, 41 retail clinics, employing 200 nurse practitioners, have opened up in Pennsylvania; these facilities are open seven days a week and have saved an estimated 150,000 emergency room visits, said Rendell.

To make affordable health care available to all children, Pennsylvania has expanded the Children's Health Insurance Program (CHIP) in an effort called Cover All Kids to provide coverage for families at higher income levels than are usually included in the program. "That is the way to expand access and make sure that the health care delivery system can be more and more affordable," said Rendell.

Under Prescription for Pennsylvania, the state also has enacted what Rendell called "the toughest health care infection law in the nation," which includes no longer paying for hospital-acquired infections through Medicaid, implementation of quality management and error reducing systems, and reporting mandates for hospital-acquired infections. These infections used to cause an estimated 3,500 deaths a year in the state and extend the hospital stays of an additional 22,000 patients. These extended hospital stays increase the average cost per patient from $35,000 to about $150,000. During the first 5 months after the law was passed, hospital-acquired infections were reduced 7.8 percent, saving $328 million, said Rendell. In addition, Rendell noted that Pennsylvania has ceased paying through Medicaid for so-called never events—medical mistakes that should never have happened, such as amputation of the wrong limb. Pennsylvania also passed a law prohibiting health care providers from billing for never events. Avoiding such medical mistakes is another way to control costs in the health care delivery system.

In 2006, 70 percent of seniors or other people living with disabilities were being treated in nursing homes across the state. With the help of nurse practitioners and physician assistants, the state has cut that number to 60 percent, said Rendell. A critical step in accomplishing this improvement was reducing barriers to practice. For example, in Pennsylvania, nurse practitioners and physician assistants previously could not do such things as order medical equipment, make physical therapy and dietician referrals, order respiratory or occupational therapy, or make general referrals. Reducing barriers to practice was also critical for certified nurse midwives. Until state laws were changed, Pennsylvania was the only state in the nation where certified nurse midwives could not prescribe drugs for their patients, even though 10 percent of all babies in the state are delivered by certified nurse midwives and in some areas they are the only source of prenatal and gynecological care.

The state also has reformed its approach to chronic care, which accounts for 80 percent of all health care costs in hospitalizations, 76 percent of all physician visits, and 91 percent of all filled prescriptions. In examining initiatives in other states, Pennsylvania found evidence of effectiveness in the Chronic Care Model that was developed by Edward Wagner, director of the Washington State McColl Institute for Healthcare Innovation. This model emphasizes managing chronic diseases through a team-based approach. "The results of this new methodology have been startling," said Rendell. Citing first-year results, Rendell noted that the number of diabetes patients who have lowered their LDL (low-density lipoprotein) cholesterol counts below 130 has increased 43 percent; the number of diabetes patients who have lowered their blood pressure below 140 over 90 has increased 25 percent; and the number of patients getting eye exams has gone up 71 percent. For diabetes in one Medicaid health maintenance organization (HMO), hospitalization costs are down 26 percent and emergency room costs are down by 18 percent during the first 10 months.

"We can do this," concluded Rendell. "Those who say that health care reform is too complicated, too difficult, . . . are dead wrong. They don't know the secret weapon, though it shouldn't be a secret much longer. The secret weapons for increasing access and increasing affordability are nurses, nurse practitioners, and physician assistants."

2

Public Policy and Public Health Nursing

The provision of community and public health nursing takes place where people live, work, and play, said Mary C. Selecky, the secretary of Washington State's Department of Health. Public health and community nurses are a part of prevention, primary care, emergency care, and long-term care across all settings, from isolated rural areas to bustling cities. This type of care involves hospitals, clinics, long-term care facilities, private providers, home and community settings, and even the media. All of these different actors and settings need to work together, which creates unique challenges for nurses.

In public health nursing, we are faced with the best of times and the worst of times, said Selecky. For example, public health nurses have collaborated at federal, state, and local levels across the country and across boundaries to play an essential role in addressing the H1N1 flu pandemic. Nurses also are working together to lead vaccination efforts and communication campaigns to promote hand washing and social distancing when people are sick. "Issues in Maine are also the issues in Washington," said Selecky. "We all touch each other because of travel."

Yet public health nursing has suffered serious setbacks recently due to economic and budget challenges across the nation. The State of Alaska has reduced public health nursing for family planning and community outreach. Connecticut has cut back the loan forgiveness program for nursing students. Florida has eliminated school nurse programs. Iowa and Maine have reduced public health nursing, and Massachusetts has eliminated the nurse's aide scholarship program. In Washington State, 300 public health positions, many filled by nurses, have been eliminated.

"Public health nursing is very complex," Selecky said, "because you take all of your clinical skills and you have to broaden them and look across the community." The Initiative on the Future of Nursing is being conducted at a critical time, said Selecky, because there will be fewer public health nurses in the future and they will face increasingly complicated problems. What kinds of skills and abilities will they need and what kinds of collaboration and partnerships will they have to forge to meet the challenges they face?

CHALLENGES FACING PUBLIC HEALTH NURSES

Selecky provided an inventory of principles that are important in public health nursing and posed a series of questions on how to better prepare public health nurses. First is a *focus on community*. Public health nurses are charged with improving the overall health of people in the community. Yet a comprehensive definition of community health takes into account healthy foods, physical activity, smoke-free homes and public places, and healthy environments. How can nurses be prepared to take on these broad policy challenges, she asked, in addition to helping sick people and managing clinical interventions?

Partnerships are essential for successful public health nursing. The governmental public health system is not solely responsible for ensuring public health. It has to work with many partners to achieve its objectives, including other parts of the health care system, Native American tribes, schools, social service agencies, environmental organizations, businesses, emergency management agencies, and homeland security. Establishing, maintaining, and strengthening these partnerships require particular skill. What kinds of skills do nurses have to acquire to foster team-based approaches to complex issues and handle limited-budget situations, and how do they acquire those skills?

Public health nurses need to draw to a much greater extent on *evidence-based prevention strategies*. An example is the community health program, Nurse-Family Partnership, that was developed by David Olds, director of the Prevention Research Center for Family and Child Health at the University of Colorado Health Sciences Center. Rigorous research has shown that the program generates substantial returns through interventions in the lives of low-income, first-time mothers and their children (Olds et al., 2007). Nurses visit these expectant mothers during their pregnancy and during the first two years of their children's lives to teach them parenting and life skills and help them gain access to job training and education. Where the Nurse-Family Partnership program was instituted in 10 counties across Washington State, for example, 90 percent of babies were born full term, 88 percent were fully immunized by 24 months, 86 percent of children had no visits to the emergency room in their first year of life due to injury or ingestion, and 93 percent of mothers initiated breast-feeding. Additionally, the program has been shown to save four dollars for every one that is invested (Karoly et al., 1998). "The Nurse-Family Partnership program has an evidence base," said Selecky. "We need to stick with that. What we have to do is let some non-evidence-based programs go."

Another example of the use of evidence to promote successful public health nursing involves school nurses. School nurses have a diverse and challenging job, and the health conditions being dealt with among student populations are increasingly complex, Selecky observed. In the Kent School District south of Seattle, 10 years ago there were 35 diabetic students and 215 students with life-threatening allergies. Today there are more than 150 diabetic students and 2,500 students with life-threatening allergies. A research review conducted by Julia Dilley found a strong correlation between school health interventions and academic achievement (Dilley, 2009). "Improved student outcomes result where schools have full-time school nurses," said Selecky.

Nurses need to be fluent in *technology*. That means much more than following someone on Twitter or being competent with a BlackBerry or a computer. It involves such tasks as retrieving data, sharing information, and mining health charts for information about both patients and the community. Programs that educate nurses need to emphasize technology and how to use it not only to communicate but also to plan, provide, and evaluate care.

Nurses also need to understand the *social determinants of health and recognize the importance of equity*, said Selecky. The demographics of communities are changing rapidly. Washington State, for example, has 29 federally recognized Native American tribes, a high percentage of Asian-American residents, and a wide range of immigrant communities. The Seattle School District routinely translates information into 40 languages. Income levels vary widely, even in areas with high average incomes. Dealing with income inequities requires an emphasis on community, especially when also working with people who speak English as a second language. Public health nurses sometimes double as health navigators to get people in the community the right information to help them make decisions for themselves, which can be further complicated when facing language and cultural differences.

Public health nursing has entered an era of *accountability and quality improvement*, Selecky said. A national movement for voluntary accreditation has placed new demands on nurses and public health agencies. In addition, nurses, more than ever, need to be skilled at *written and verbal communication*. Nurses may be skilled at interacting with patients, but they also need to be able to write clearly and speak in front of groups to influence and effectively improve the health of people in their communities.

Public health nurses must have mastered *the basics of their professions*. They must promote immunization, detect emergency health threats, and prevent and respond to communicable diseases. In addition, they need to be prepared to deal with *public health emergencies*. For example, an increasing number of nurses need to be trained in incident command. Selecky works closely with the chief of the state police patrol and the adjutant general of the National Guard, as well as the head of the department of social and health services. In 2007 when the town of Chehalis south of Seattle experienced one of the worst floods in 100 years, a public health nurse called Selecky to ask how to deal with and dispose of dead cows, an unforeseen challenge as a public health nurse. The nurse knew she needed tetanus shots and portable toilets but had not anticipated other, less common, aspects of the emergency. "We all have to learn to deal with emergencies, no matter what they are," said Selecky.

PUBLIC POLICY IMPLICATIONS

Ensuring public health has important implications for the involvement of nurses in public policy, said Selecky. First, public health cannot be separated from politics. Politics is part of everything public health nurses do, as demonstrated by the term "public." Intrinsically, politics need not always have a negative connotation—it consists of the art and science of government and governing. Similarly, while some may view politicians negatively, they are not inherently devious; they are public servants elected to represent the values and beliefs of their constituents, noted Selecky.

Second, science is not policy, but science informs the development of policy. Community values also inform public policy, which again emphasizes the importance of communication and relationships. In addition, political instinct and judgment are essential skills for public health nurses to master. For that reason, public health leaders, including nurses, must have well-honed strategy skills. They must know the public health needs of their communities and understand the science and the best policy and implementation options for meeting community needs and values. Public health leaders and nurses need to provide a buffer and a bridge between the political world and the health world. Larry Wallack, dean of Portland State University's College of Urban and Public Affairs, once said, "I have never heard data say a word. It is people who take it and turn it into information for other people." Selecky asked, "Who can do that better than a nurse? Who is best trusted when there is a tough health issue? A nurse." Nurses need to understand their role in the development and implementation of public policies that impact health. They also need to inform public policy with science and evidence-based facts and be ethical, professional, and collaborative, said Selecky.

The third point Selecky highlighted is that the current investment in public health does not meet the need at a time when all expenditures are being scrutinized. Washington and many other states are facing severe budget deficits, which means that every dollar spent has to be examined. "My budget is 50 percent federal dollars and only 20 percent state general funds, but every one of those [dollars] is essential." Accountability and performance requirements are increasing, which means that evidence-based practices will be further emphasized.

Selecky notes that nurses' roles, in general, will continue to be essential, regardless of what happens with health care reform. Nurses affect access, affordability, and health care improvement and are the best teachers in the health care system. They need to understand politics, public health, and partnerships. They have to be comfortable with new technologies and talk plainly and clearly, said Selecky. They need to know the basics of public health and be prepared for new health threats, changing priorities, and new opportunities.

Selecky concluded by offering the committee three suggestions pertaining to the education and professional development of all nurses:

1. The nursing curriculum needs to change to focus on policy, technology, and community-based practice. "No matter if you are in an institution or working in a hospice or in a governmental or for-profit organization, if you are a nurse you need to understand your impact on the community," said Selecky.
2. Schools of nursing need to place considerable emphasis on verbal and written communications. They also need to graduate life-

      long learners who have the ability to learn new things and change course along the way.

3. Nurses need leadership development programs, particularly in community settings.

RESPONSES TO QUESTIONS

In response to a question about the need to diversify the public health nursing workforce, Selecky responded that it is absolutely essential. In Washington State, she participated in hearings across the state in minority communities to discuss opportunities in the health professions. Many students at those hearings recounted how they became interested in science. For example, a teacher expressed an interest in a student, a student was inspired by a role model, or a student was invited to attend an after-school science club. "I challenge every one of you to find your replacement. Talk to somebody you didn't talk to before. Go into a different place in your community and say, 'Are there any kids who might want to talk to me and find out what it is like to be a nurse?' Because they may never have had that opportunity. You are part of the solution," stressed Selecky.

Augmenting the preparation of nurses may require involving people from other parts of a university or college, such as a faculty member in political science, public policy, or communications. At the University of Washington's School of Public Health, Selecky's communications director often talks with students. "He shows clips from bad interviews and clips from good interviews and [describes] what you can learn and how you can handle that situation differently. You don't have to have the same person doing the same thing to be able to expand the curriculum," said Selecky.

In addition, many valuable written materials are available about public health and its connection with public policy, such as the Institute of Medicine's 1988 and 2002 reports on public health (IOM, 1988, 2002). Selecky said that "there is a lot of learning for us to do, [but] there are a lot of resources to build on."

A member of the audience asked about the role of public health nurses in community evaluations and interventions, and Selecky responded that she would like to have nurses represented in many state divisions, such as the division of environmental health. Nurses could look at issues such as asthma, which is common in Washington State.

"Nurses bring incredible diagnostic skills—what in some [contexts] is called community assessment," Selecky said. On home visits, nurses can pay attention not just to an infant but to whether the house is littered with garbage, whether a father is present, or whether there is food in the kitchen. "The nurse of the future will have those skills."

A question from someone watching the webcast of the forum asked about improving health beyond the bedside and in the community, and Selecky described two women who received associate degrees in nursing when she was working in a rural area of Washington State. When the women asked her whether she had jobs for them, she put them both to work knowing that nurses interested in public and community health are often swept up into acute care, where most jobs for nurses are. "Did they have all the community nursing experience that you might want them to have? No. But that was my job, to make sure that they got that type of experience and training and oversight," said Selecky.

Selecky also was asked about the intersection between public health nursing and mental health. "We are whole bodies and whole communities," she responded, yet the mental health system is often in a separate silo from public health nursing, partly because of how the two kinds of services are funded. "Perhaps we need to have public health nurses embedded within our mental health system, and vice versa," she suggested.

3

Community and Public Health

NURSING IN THE COMMUNITY

Carol Raphael, president and CEO of the Visiting Nurse Service of New York (VNSNY), described the work of VNSNY, its nursing workforce, and how technology is used to support its workforce. VNSNY is the largest nonprofit home health care agency in the United States; it was founded in 1893 by Lillian Wald and serves all five boroughs of New York City plus Westchester and Nassau counties. Every day VNSNY provides a range of services to a case population of approximately 30,000, from newborns to seniors, and about 2,600 nurses are among its 14,000 employees.

The VNSNY has a complex patient population to whom it provides a wide range of programs and services. These programs and services fall roughly into three categories. The first category is preventive care, including care provided for patients in congregate care facilities.[1] The second category is home-based care, including post-acute care, long-term care, and hospice and palliative care. The VNSNY also functions as a health plan payer through a Medicaid Managed Long-Term Care program and through a Medicare Advantage Special Needs Plan.

Raphael described the average patients that VNSNY serves. The most common diagnoses among VNSNY's patients are chronic conditions, including diabetes, hypertension, and congestive heart failure

---

[1]Congregate care facilities are residential settings that typically provide social activities, security, and assistance with instrumental activities of daily living (e.g., meal preparation, housekeeping, transportation). Residents tend to have health care needs that fall between those of individuals who live independently in the community and those of individuals who require the health services of an assisted living facility or nursing home.

(CHF). These diagnoses occur with an average of four other conditions; some common co-occurring diagnoses are CHF and chronic obstructive pulmonary disease (COPD); CHF and diabetes; and hypertension and dementia. On average, patients take eight different medications. About 9 percent have cognitive impairments, and 16 percent have a history of diagnosed depression or self-reported symptoms of depression—a figure that is likely an underestimate of the true proportion of cases suffering from depression. They usually have impairments in five to six ADLs (activities of daily living). About 50 to 75 percent of patients are from minority groups, and at least 36 different languages are spoken across VNSNY's patient population.

The nurses who provide care through the VNSNY "have to do it all," said Raphael. "They are the admissions office. They have to do the financial eligibility. We say, 'When we walk into a home, we walk into a life.' Our second major reason for worker's compensation claims among our nurses is dog bites.[2] You never know what you are going to face when you walk into someone's home."

The role of the VNSNY nurse varies depending on the setting and the needs of the patients. In congregate care, the role of the onsite nurse is threefold:

1. To conduct health promotion and education activities for residents, families, and building staff.
2. To provide case management for residents who need ongoing support for chronic conditions and to provide linkages to community resources.
3. To screen, assess, and link residents to home health care as needed.

For home care patients, the coordination of interdisciplinary care is a critical function of visiting nurses. They help patients recover and regain functioning, learn to manage their own conditions, avoid exacerbations in chronic conditions, and build up strength and endurance. This can encompass a wide range of nursing roles. Nurses may assess needs, the home environment, and financial coverage; develop and implement a plan of care; facilitate communication between and among providers and patients; document progress; manage medications; monitor for declines;

---

[2]The first major cause for worker's compensations claims among VNSNY nurses is "slips, trips, and falls," which can happen anywhere the nurses go (e.g., sidewalks, offices, or clients homes) but incidents most often occur on stairs.

intervene before crises; and establish appropriate follow-up care or transfers to a different program.

Raphael cited examples of transitional care models developed by Mary Naylor, director of NewCourtland Center for Transitions and Health at the University of Pennsylvania School of Nursing, and Eric Coleman, professor of medicine at the University of Colorado. Using these models, nurses ensure that appropriate steps have occurred within the first 30 days of home care, a critical period of time when 16 percent of home health episodes result in hospitalization (Meadow, 2007). Following discharge, as many as 34 percent of patients may return to the hospital within 90 days of discharge, as a recent study involving Medicare fee-for-service patients found (Jencks et al., 2009). Nurses using transitional care models evaluate the risk of rehospitalization, develop emergency response plans, reconcile and simplify medications, make follow-up appointments with community providers, and plan for discharge from home care. Patients have an "action plan" that sets goals and responsibilities. This plan is posted in the home so that the patient will call VNSNY rather than 9-1-1 when there is a problem. In the 2 years since VNSNY started implementing transitional care, the rehospitalization rate of home care patients dropped from 27 percent to 23.5 percent, said Raphael.

VNSNY also operates a Nurse-Family Partnership program, such as the one described by Mary Selecky in Chapter 2, that ensures prenatal care; educates prospective parents about newborn care; fosters the physical, emotional, and cognitive development of children; and links families to other community supports and programs. The Father's First program has been interlaced with the Nurse-Family Partnership to promote the increased involvement of fathers in parenting.

VNSNY operates two health plans programs specific to Medicaid and Medicare populations. In the Medicaid Managed Long-Term Care plan, nurses support plan members in the community, help to avoid nursing home stays, and manage members across settings. In the Medicare Advantage Special Needs Plan, nurses help members avoid preventable hospital and emergency room visits by ensuring the provision of primary care and by addressing service gaps. Special attention, including increased follow-up and additional communication and case management, is focused on the 15 percent of patients who are considered highest risk. "So far we are seeing considerable success," said Raphael. "We devote a far lower portion of our premium to in-patient hospital stays than comparable Medicare Advantage plans do."

Technology Supports for Nurses

Technology is a central component of VNSNY operations, said Raphael. All of its clinicians use laptops equipped with proprietary structured electronic health records. The clinician synchronizes the laptop with the VNSNY network from the field and is able to retrieve current data at the point of care. The technology was adapted by studying systems for mobile workforces, such as those used by Federal Express and other field-based organizations. "It is inconceivable that we could function without this system, which was further designed and developed by our nurses," said Raphael. The technology has been universally adopted by the staff, so much so that any interruptions in service generate an immediate reaction.

Information in the mobile system is evidence-based, which forces providers to think about how their actions apply to different chronic conditions. The system also generates quality measures based on outcomes, processes, satisfaction, and utilization, with each care team receiving its quality results. "[Providers] can go to the website and retrieve [the results] and see how they are doing compared to every other team." An arrangement with the unions representing workers allowed a test of linking pay to quality results. "It is 'walking the talk' and showing that this does in fact matter in terms of what we evaluate and value," said Raphael.

The technology has also enabled information exchanges with hospitals and physicians. For example, pilot programs with several large physician groups are evaluating the exchange in real time of information about patients shared in common. Raphael said, "That will really be a breakthrough for us in terms of changing how we think about what we do."

The Evolving Roles of Nurses

The roles of nurses at the VNSNY have evolved from being task-oriented and transactional to being outcomes-oriented and relational. Nurses used to have short-term relationships with patients; when they changed a wound dressing, they did it alone; and payments were tied to fee-for-service systems and volume. Now, the system has shifted to an emphasis on outcomes over extended periods, such as the ability to regain function, prevent complications and decline, and maintain a good quality of life. Nurses are the coordinators of interdisciplinary teams that can include physical, occupational, and speech therapists; social workers; family and other informal caregivers; physicians; and pharmacists. Raphael recalled, "One of the nurses said to me, 'It used to be about me. Now, it is about the patient.'"

Raphael identified six skills that community health nurses will need in the future. Nurses need the ability to

1. Assess risk levels, functional impairments, and the medical and support needs of individuals;
2. Partner with the patient and the patient's family to develop a reasonable and achievable plan of care;
3. Manage a cross-disciplinary team, including informal caregivers;
4. Coordinate care with other providers across settings;
5. Aggregate, synthesize, interpret, and act on clinical data; and
6. Communicate effectively with patients and caregiving teams.

The need for these skills has many implications for nursing education, in which VNSNY plays an active role. A nurse internship program offers new bachelor's degree nursing graduates hands-on experience and mentoring by seasoned staff to prepare them for home-based nursing. Thirty members of the nursing staff are adjunct faculty at nursing schools. About 500 nursing students come through VNSNY on clinical rotations each year, but much of the education and training for VNSNY nurses still occurs on the job. "We really have to do a lot of our own education and training to compensate for the fact that most of the nurses don't come with the experience, the competencies, or the comfort and confidence with technology that we think they need," Raphael concluded.

THE FUTURE OF NURSES IN COMMUNITY CARE

Dr. Eileen Sullivan-Marx, the associate dean for practice and community affairs at the University of Pennsylvania School of Nursing, recently chaired a commission in Pennsylvania on the future of senior care services and resources in the state. As the only nurse on the commission, she applied a lesson well known among nurses: "Hearing from the public is an important piece to get you to that next step."

Within the context of senior care services, the commission examined the current state of nursing, data about its future, and where the profession is headed. Yet understanding nursing also requires understanding the passion of the individuals in the profession. "This is particularly important with students," Sullivan-Marx said. "Students often resonate with different images of nursing than do members of older generations."

Attracting people to community nursing requires social marketing, including discussion of price, place, promotion, and positioning. Working in the community has to be an attractive career track for nurses, and it has to have social and financial returns comparable to the investments made in the profession and to other career paths that nurses can pursue. Communities need to be accessible, and target audiences need to be made aware of what community nurses do.

Nurses are among the most trusted professionals in the United States, Sullivan-Marx said. Yet community nursing usually remains invisible in the broader society. Community nurses need to position themselves to have maximum benefits and minimal costs if the profession is to remain viable.

The Health Resources and Services Administration (HRSA) has studied the projected supply, demand, and shortages of nurses up to 2020 (HRSA, 2004b) and has found that the projected demand for registered nurses will rise most quickly for nurses working in the community; see Table 3-1 and Table 3-2. "We are still thinking much more about workforce shortages in hospitals, and, yes, that is where it is acute. But look where the real projected demand is . . . in home health care, with community care beyond that," said Sullivan-Marx.

TABLE 3-1 National Measures of Projected Nurse Staffing Intensity

Setting	Staff Intensity	2000	2010	2020	Increase in Demand 2000-2020
Short-term hospital (inpatient)	RNs per 1,000 patient-days	6.54	7.12	7.69	18%
Long-term hospital	RNs per 1,000 patient-days	5.25	5.29	5.27	0%
Nursing facility	RNs per resident	0.10	0.11	0.11	13%
Home health	RNs per 1,000 visits	2.87	3.31	3.84	34%

NOTES: RN = registered nurse. This table demonstrates projected demand at the national level using baseline assumptions defined for HRSA's Nursing Demand Model. However, demand at the state level varies significantly. HRSA also reports alternate national scenarios based on changes in model assumptions (e.g., RN wage increase, greater population growth) and methodological information.
SOURCE: HRSA (2004b).

TABLE 3-2 Projected Demand for FTE RNs

Setting	FTE RNs 2000	FTE RNs 2010	FTE RNs 2020	Increase in Demand 2000-2020
Short-term hospital (inpatient)	874,000	999,100	1,187,000	36%
Long-term hospital	191,000	223,900	269,400	41%
Nursing facility	172,800	224,500	287,300	66%
Home health	132,000	187,500	275,600	109%

NOTES: FTE = full-time equivalent; RN = registered nurse. This table demonstrates projected demand at the national level using baseline assumptions defined for HRSA's Nursing Demand Model. However, demand at the state level varies significantly. HRSA also reports alternate national scenarios based on changes in model assumptions (e.g., RN wage increase, greater population growth) and methodological information.
SOURCE: HRSA (2004b).

Sullivan-Marx offered seven recommendations for the committee when considering the future of home, community, and public health nursing:

1. *Establish professional nursing roles in places where people live and work.* Students need to learn and seek jobs in these settings. For example, Sullivan-Marx tries to get her students into health fairs and other activities in the community. However, there are not enough opportunities for students to gain experience in the community.
2. *Maximize benefits and minimize costs.* This requires reframing care not by place but by skills and services. Skills should not be limited to a particular setting. "We are still too much bound by settings and how we think about payment structures and where nurses go," said Sullivan-Marx
3. *Enable nurses to control practice.* Payment for nursing services needs to be visible, transparent, fair, and based on outcome incentives. Sullivan-Marx said, "Payment is the recognition of our authority to practice by society."
4. *Foster and recognize independent decision making by basic and advanced practice nurses.* Although progress has been made in this area, many problems remain. For example, Sullivan-Marx noted that changes in Pennsylvania have enabled nurses to order

durable medical equipment, but by federal statute they cannot do so if the equipment is paid for by Medicare.

5. *Establish quality in community care as a core competency for all nurses.* Patient safety considerations extend far beyond the boundaries of hospitals, and the core competencies taught in nursing schools should reflect that fact.

6. *Embrace family- and patient-centered care with a team of providers with nurses as leaders in care.*

7. Finally, *lead the return and renewal of public health nursing.*

RESPONSES TO QUESTIONS

In response to a question about recruiting and retaining nurses, Raphael noted that the VNSNY "had a very difficult time in recruitment" until about a year and a half ago. Before that, VNSNY paid sign-on bonuses, but nurses tended to come for one year and then leave to get a sign-on bonus elsewhere. In response, the organization decided to focus special attention on retention. Raphael noted that all new employees have a mentor who keeps in touch regularly. Efforts are made not to overwhelm new employees and to address any issues early. Because the staff works in the field, VNSNY tries to establish social networks to increase interactions. As a result of these efforts, Raphael said that VNSNY now has just a 2 percent vacancy rate among nurses in its certified home health agency.

VNSNY also has had difficulties recruiting staff from diverse communities. About 20 percent of its patients are Hispanic, but less than 2 percent of nurses in the United States are Hispanic, "so there is a mismatch in the pool," said Raphael. Some nurses are going to a Berlitz course to learn Spanish, while others travel with translators. Raphael also said that at one point, VNSNY had many Korean patients but virtually no Korean nurses. Finally, by recruiting one Korean nurse, they were able to make contact with others, and now they have 29 Korean nurses. "Recruitment efforts have been completely through the community."

Sullivan-Marx noted that retention also has improved in a comprehensive program of full-time interdisciplinary care with which she is involved—from more than 30 percent turnover several years ago to about 5 percent. "The reason our folks stay . . . is because they feel they are making a difference. They also have benefits that we are able to offer through the university," including opportunities for continuing education, said Sullivan-Marx. One factor behind retention is that staff feel they are contributing to the communities where they were raised. "Many people say, 'This woman was my teacher. I feel like I am giving her the best care that I could possibly give.'"

Sullivan-Marx added that recruiting new, young nurses directly from school is more difficult because they may not have the ability to "jump in and do the independent, critical thinking that is required in community care." They may struggle with their roles and what is expected of them.

Raphael said that her organization has attracted people from other fields, such as financial services or the media, who are interested in becoming nurses, but "it is not easy to make that leap." The largest source of nurses for VNSNY is the acute care setting. The organization has a 3-week orientation program for nurses from acute care or nursing homes to introduce them to community care, followed by continuing education. Raphael said, "The nurses often find it very difficult, because you don't have someone down the hall you can go to ask for advice. You are often completely autonomous, and you have to make judgment calls." Raphael described a family in which a woman with severe cancer insisted that 24 hours before she died she should be moved to a hospital so that her spirit would not remain in the family home. The new nurse was "very rattled," said Raphael. "She wanted to be sure she made this family feel comfortable. I don't think she felt 100 percent sure she was going to know 24 hours before that that was the time, though an experienced hospice nurse would have known."

There needs to be a culture shift so that nurses seek help when it is needed; community and public health nurses need to feel that they can reach out and ask for help. "You have to figure out a way to give ongoing support and help as these unexpected issues emerge," Raphael said. Sullivan-Marx emphasized the importance of mentorship programs to support and educate nurses new to community care.

Sullivan-Marx noted during her talk that nursing cannot remain a largely female profession. "We are not going to be able to meet the demand." Raphael observed that VNSNY has had success recruiting males from fire departments and the military. "People have worked for 20 to 25 years. They are in their forties, and now they want a second career," noted Raphael. As a result of targeted recruitment, her organization has a higher percentage of men in the nursing workforce than is the case elsewhere.

In response to a question about technologies that could help community nursing, Raphael mentioned remote patient monitoring and the evaluation of so-called smart homes that use sensors placed throughout the home to monitor patients' mobility, medication use, and potential problems. This technology creates a different role for nurses, who have to interpret information remotely and determine when someone needs a visit from a caregiver. "Some of the nurses are welcoming that role, and this is a technology we are looking at seriously." She also said that VNSNY nurses often take photographs of wounds and show the photographs to wound care specialists and physicians to determine if a therapy needs to be changed. "One of the most important things we can do is link with the primary care physician and be able to exchange clinical information on a continuous basis," she noted.

Sullivan-Marx also cited the potential for technologies to maintain communication between patients and nurses. For example, family caregivers may need to access information from nurses 24 hours a day. Technologies that can provide information quickly and easily would be welcomed by these families.

4

Primary Care

NURSE PRACTITIONERS AS LEADERS IN PRIMARY CARE

Having access to health insurance does not necessarily mean having access to primary care services or access to high-quality, efficient health care, said Tine Hansen-Turton, the CEO of the National Nursing Centers Consortium and executive director of the Convenient Care Association. For example, when the Commonwealth of Massachusetts passed health care reform legislation in 2007, more than 300,000 people got a new insurance card. However, emergency rooms were immediately flooded with patients, and physicians' offices had to quit accepting new patients because of the overwhelming demand. "We learned some very important lessons from Massachusetts," said Hansen-Turton—one of which is that the nursing workforce needs to be prepared and empowered to deliver primary care. Nurse practitioners are "ready, willing, and able to be primary care providers and a partner in this crisis," she said.

The State of Pennsylvania has devoted considerable attention to the development and use of the nursing workforce. For example, legislation has expanded the scope of practice for nurses and has reduced some of the barriers for nurse practitioners and other clinical nurse specialists to practice to their greatest potential in the state (Hansen-Turton et al., 2009). The state also has invested in the Chronic Care Model that Governor Rendell described during his remarks; as he noted, this model uses nurse practitioners and primary care physicians in a medical home format to reach three-quarters of a million patients.

Nurse-Managed Health Clinics

Another important way to provide health care, particularly to vulnerable populations, is through nurse-managed health clinics. Today there are about 250 such clinics in the United States, and "we hope there will be many more in the future," said Hansen-Turton. These clinics are staffed by nurse practitioners, other advanced practice nurses, registered nurses, therapists and social workers, midwives, outreach workers, psychologists, collaborating physicians, health educators, students, administrative personnel, and other health professionals. They are located where people are—in shopping malls, in community centers, and sometimes in mobile vans. They generally offer low-cost, high-quality, community-based primary care and behavioral health, prenatal, and wellness services; some also offer dentistry and mental health services. About one-third are independent nonprofits, and two-thirds are affiliated with academic institutions, which enables these clinics to act as training sites for nurses and nursing students.

Approximately 46 percent of the patients seen at nurse-managed health clinics are uninsured, and 37 percent are on Medicaid. "You can't sustain a business model on that unless you get grant funding, . . . so that is a challenge," noted Hansen-Turton. However, the average primary care cost for these clinics is 10 percent less than for other types of providers, and the average personnel cost is 11 percent less than other providers' costs. For patients who use these clinics, emergency room use, hospitalization, maternity days, specialty care costs, and prescription costs are all lower, she said. Yet nurse-managed health clinics see their members an average of 1.8 times more than other providers, and patients report high satisfaction with the care they receive at the clinics (Hansen-Turton et al., 2004).

Nurse-managed health clinics face a number of challenges, said Hansen-Turton. One is the patchwork of funding on which they rely—a combination of inconsistent reimbursement, federal dollars, and state and local funding. "The real issue is that the health care system has not quite caught up to the innovation of these clinics." A recent national survey found that nearly half of all major managed care organizations do not credential or contract with nurse practitioners as primary care providers (Hansen-Turton et al., 2008). "That is going to be an issue if we want to avoid what is going on and what went on in Massachusetts when we get health insurance reform," said Hansen-Turton.

The National Center on Quality Assurance (NCQA), which administers a certification program to recognize patient-centered medical homes, has said that its certification can be used only to accredit physician-led practices. Also, nurse practitioners cannot currently participate in some of the medical home initiatives supported by the Centers for Medicare & Medicaid Services. Very recently, however, the Joint Commission, a nationwide accrediting body for health care organizations across a variety of settings, has approved certification for a primary care home that includes nurse practitioners and physician assistants in leadership roles. Hansen-Turton said, "I think NCQA eventually will change, but it is important because certification is tied into reimbursement."

Convenient Care Clinics

Another way to increase access to cost-effective care is through retail-based convenient care clinics, said Hansen-Turton, of which there are now about 1,200 in the United States. Services in these clinics are provided primarily by nurse practitioners, and no appointments are necessary. The clinics typically are located in retail outlets and have retail service hours, which generally extend beyond normal office hours for physicians. Pricing is transparent, with services typically costing between $40 and $75 —significantly less than a visit to the emergency room or to a physician's office; see Figure 4-1.

Hansen-Turton noted that the clinics generally accept insurance although about 35 percent of patients choose to pay out of pocket. Some of the insurance companies have embraced this model and have waived copays because they see it as a way to alleviate pressure on emergency rooms. The clinics use electronic health records and evidence-based medicine. Hansen-Turton said that she, her husband, and their son are typical users, having gone to such clinics about eight times in the past year. "We got immunized, we had a couple of strep throats, we had some ear infections, and we were in and out in about 30 minutes. It doesn't get much better than that for those types of services," said Hansen-Turton.

Research has supported the value of convenient care clinics. It has found that the care they provide is on a par with care from primary care physicians, urgent care centers, and emergency rooms in terms of quality and cost (Mehrotra et al., 2009). They are within a 10-minute drive for one-third of all Americans (Rudavsky et al., 2009), and they are

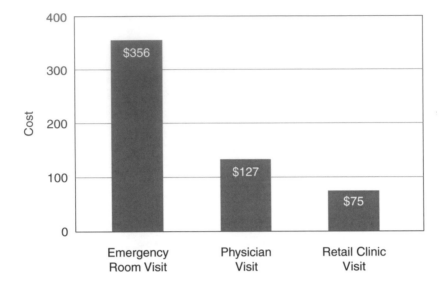

FIGURE 4-1 Comparison of costs associated with typical visits to the emergency room, physicians, and a retail clinic.
NOTE: "Typical visits" consisted of the three episodes that account for 48 percent of acute visits in retail-based convenient care clinics: otitis media, pharyngitis, and urinary tract infections.

effective in reaching the segment of the U.S. population that currently goes without regular care, with up to 60 percent of clinic patients not having a regular source of primary care (Mehrotra et al., 2008). "If you talk with any of the managed care organizations that contract with [the clinics], they'll say that this is our lowest-cost health care option," noted Hansen-Turton.

Nurse-Managed Health Clinics, Convenient Care Clinics, and Nurse Practitioners: Considerations for the Future

Hansen-Turton drew several suggestions from her overview of nurse-managed health clinics and convenient care clinics for the committee's consideration. First, she noted that these clinics demonstrate the need to support new models that broaden access to quality care: "As everybody gets an insurance card, you are going to need places where you can get care." For this reason, Hansen-Turton said that the Centers for Medicare & Medicaid Services should support medical home and performance-based demonstrations that include nurse-managed health clinics with nurse practitioners as primary care providers and convenient care clinics. Also, she said that managed care organizations and insurance companies should credential nurse practitioners as primary care providers, which would help to create an environment in which nurse practitioners and advanced practice nurses can perform all of the functions permitted under state scope-of-practice laws. Massachusetts took several of these steps after passing its health care reform legislation in 2007, and the laws passed there could be a model for states elsewhere (Craven and Ober, 2009).

In general, health care in the future will have a new focus on consumers. Hansen-Turton noted that young people in particular do not necessarily think of health care in the same way that older generations have. Customers who demand services that provide more value and are more affordable will catalyze disruptive innovations,[1] and as Lee has stated, disruption needs to be seen as a virtue (Lee and Lansky, 2008). "Continuing to allow the perpetuation of the status quo will not improve Americans' health status," concluded Hansen-Turton.

THE INDIAN HEALTH SERVICE: A RURAL HEALTH CARE SERVICE

The Indian Health Service (IHS) employs more than 4,000 registered nurses, including more than 300 advanced practice nurses. It provides health care to 1.9 million American Indians and Alaska Natives around the country, mostly on reservations in rural and remote areas. Its system includes 48 hospitals; several hundred ambulatory, free-standing primary care clinics; and 34 urban clinics. Under Indian self-determination, about half of the service's programs are now managed and operated by tribes themselves. Sandra Haldane, the chief nurse and director of the Division of Nursing at IHS, provided an overview of its accomplishments and bar-

---

[1]A "disruptive innovation" has been defined by Clayton Christensen as "a process by which a product or service takes root initially in simple applications at the bottom of a market and then relentlessly moves 'up market,' eventually displacing established competitors. An innovation that is disruptive allows a whole new population of consumers access to a product or service that was historically only accessible to consumers with a lot of money or a lot of skill" (Christensen, 1997, 2009).

riers to progress and offered the committee suggestions to convert challenges into achievements.

Most of IHS's nurse practitioners are family nurse practitioners functioning as licensed independent practitioners under federal scope-of-practice guidelines. In the primary care setting, nurse practitioners have their own panels of patients, see a full load on a daily basis, and travel several times a week to satellite clinics and schools. They offer women's health and midwifery services, pediatrics and well-child care, care for elders, and interventions for psychiatric and mental health conditions.

In recent years, the service has recognized that it is ill prepared and understaffed to deal with the high rates of sexual assault and domestic violence in the communities it serves. "In almost every instance, it has been nurse practitioners and nurse midwives who have taken on this issue," said Haldane. They have become forensic experts and medical examiners and have worked with community partners to form programs so that people do not have to travel hours to get to private sector facilities for needed services. Haldane said that in the past 2 years, IHS has trained 60 forensic nurse examiners. Additionally, facilities have established programs to screen for sexually transmitted diseases, organized programs to facilitate mother-daughter interactions, and held faculty dinners at the high school and middle school levels to educate community leaders and youth on healthy lifestyles, behaviors, and risk factors.

IHS includes more than 350 public health nurses prepared at the bachelor's level who are rarely found in clinics and hospitals but rather are out in the community. "They can be found making home visits to patients who have missed important appointments, checking on patients after discharges, or assisting with dressing changes in the home," said Haldane. "They can be found assessing the safety of our elders' homes, doing developmental testing of children at risk, going into reservation correctional facilities to provide screening and also into schools for health education, screening, well-child checks, and immunizations. They can be found at fitness centers, sports tournaments, concerts, and pulling over to the side of the road to visit with our Indian arts and crafts vendors to administer flu vaccine," she said. This group of nurses is often the first to notice a change in disease patterns in the community that could indicate an infectious outbreak, as occurred recently when the public health nursing program at a facility in the southwestern region recognized a steady increase in gastrointestinal events as signaling an outbreak of salmonella.

Many advanced practice nurses and public health nurses in IHS have helped increase access to care and reduce disparities. Haldane described a program in Anchorage that was born out of a need to reduce the high rate of infant mortality in the native population there. All mothers were screened for risk factors, and those at risk were followed for a year, with nurses providing in-home education on growth and development, safety and nutrition education, immunizations, and referral to other community services. "The results have been outstanding," said Haldane. Over a 5-year period the average number of days between infant deaths went from 55 to 130, the targeted population had decreased hospital admissions, the time between pregnancies increased, the use of emergency rooms fell, identified maltreatment declined, and more mothers appeared to be staying clean and sober.

Another example that Haldane cited is a reservation the size of Connecticut, on the border of Arizona and New Mexico, with 14,000 tribal members. In early 2007 the number of reported cases of syphilis increased dramatically to approximately three to five cases per month. Public health nurses worked with the tribe and parents to decrease the stigma of sexually transmitted diseases and get students to consent to screening. They developed culturally appropriate educational materials and took these materials into community centers and concerts. They conducted door-to-door campaigns to offer on-the-spot screening in a manner that would not embarrass tribal members or risk offense to tribal standards. The rate of new syphilis cases dropped significantly in 2008, and in the first part of 2009 there were no documented cases, said Haldane.

In some American Indian cultures it is not appropriate to talk about disasters, especially in the context of the future, so when a public health nurse on the Navajo Reservation began exploring ways to work with other preparedness entities, she had to do so without offending a very traditional people. "Through her insight and keen talent for relationship building, this public health nurse and her team developed a mass vaccination campaign to avert a disaster," said Haldane. Community clinics were established and staffed with medical personnel as well as community volunteers so that they could work together to address threats in a community-based way.

Public health nurses must cover a broad spectrum of health concerns within the populations and communities they serve. Haldane observed that type 2 diabetes and obesity have become widespread, pressing problems among American Indian youth. In one community a public health nurse who is also an avid soccer father worked to bring the American Youth Soccer Organization to the community, which gave Navajo children a fun and different physical activity they had not had access to previously.

Challenges for the Indian Health Service

Most IHS facilities are not rural; they are considered frontier,[2] which brings a distinctive set of recruitment, retention, and practice challenges. The service's vacancy rate for nurses in 2008 was 21 percent. In 2009, however, the vacancy rate decreased to 18 percent, perhaps because more nurses returned to the workforce as the economy weakened, said Haldane. Advanced practice nurses working within the IHS system still face some prejudice from physicians, who have a tendency to say that their patients are too complex for advanced practice nurses and more doctors need to be hired. Haldane also noted that more and more public health nursing programs are being cut because the majority of states do not reimburse services provided by public health nurses. IHS is authorized to spend only a certain amount on loan repayment for nurses, and advanced practice nurses have to compete with physician assistants for the same pool of loan repayment funds. "Thus, every year we end up with a significant number of advanced practice nurses who are matched to sites that qualify for loan repayment but do not get it because we run out of funds," said Haldane.

The primary reason that 60 percent of the IHS's registered nursing workforce is American Indian and Alaskan Native is because of a scholarship program available through IHS. However, of the hundreds of applications received each year, only about 100 students can be funded. For those who wish to go to school to achieve an advanced practice degree, opportunities are "dismal," according to Haldane. The service's system is seeing continuous decline in inpatient admissions and an increasing use of primary care and public health services, yet most new nurses' education has focused on inpatient nursing. Indeed, some schools have dramatically curtailed their community and public health work because of

---

[2]The Rural Assistance Center describes frontier areas as "the most rural settled places along the rural-urban continuum, with residents far from health care, schools, grocery stores, and other necessities. Frontier is often thought of in terms of population density and distance in minutes and miles to population centers and other resources, such as hospitals" (http://www.raconline.org/info_guides/frontier).

student safety issues—thus producing students even less prepared for this type of work, said Haldane.

The population served by IHS tends to equate health care with physicians. "We struggle daily with how to educate our people on the advantages of advanced practice nurses," said Haldane. "We struggle with awareness of what advanced practice nurses can do and with administrators who [mistakenly] believe that a nurse is a nurse is a nurse.... I can only speak for the Indian Health Service, but I doubt that these issues are exclusive to us," said Haldane.

Despite the pressures of cost containment, it has to be possible to reimburse public health nursing activities such as going into high-risk homes to provide immunizations or to assess the growth and development of at-risk infants, said Haldane. Commissions, committees, and other entities tend to focus on health care that takes place in metropolitan and urban areas. More resources need to be focused on the health care system and the types of nurses it takes to provide access and quality to patients living in remote, rural, and frontier locations. About 1.2 percent of the U.S. population is American Indian or Alaskan Native. Yet only 0.1 percent of the nursing workforce is of that ethnicity, Haldane said. Programs that successfully recruit and retain American Indian and Alaskan Native nursing students will yield positive outcomes for patients.

Haldane also noted that under federal Office of Personnel Management rules, nurses are not always paid for being on call, and their overtime is capped. "They feel like they are providing unpaid volunteer service," said Haldane. Changing payroll practices would help, but so would better reimbursement mechanisms so that additional staff could be hired to fill the need. Finally, the nursing profession must relentlessly educate the general public about the roles of advanced practice nurses, concluded Haldane.

RESPONSES TO QUESTIONS

A questioner asked whether retail care clinics actually save money or whether they treat health problems that might have been ignored if a clinic were not available. Hansen-Turton replied that retail clinics are not meant to be ongoing sources of primary care. However, they are designed to provide basic health care services, and emergency rooms are now being flooded with people needing attention for various types of basic health care issues that could be treated elsewhere. Since retail clinics are available to everyone and are open during extended hours, they can provide access to basic continuity of care that may not be available to some people elsewhere in the health care system. "The task is designing a system in which all the pieces fit together smoothly. The real value proposition is multiple access to care, and certainly the retail clinics present a first level of care," said Hansen-Turton.

In response to a question about how to increase the diversity of the nursing workforce and reduce barriers these candidates face in entering the nursing profession, Haldane said that many of the students who apply for scholarship programs through IHS are from remote and rural locations and are not as well prepared as other individuals. The service offers robust scholarship programs to assist qualified individuals, but it does not have enough funding for everyone who applies. Haldane also said that graduate students need adequate support and good mentors to transition from a student role into that of a fully functioning nurse.

5

Chronic and Long-Term Services and Supports

NURSES' ROLES IN MEETING LONG-TERM HEALTH CARE NEEDS

Within the next two decades, at least 20 percent of Americans will be 65 and older. Nurses must play a leadership role in caring for this population, said Dr. Claudia Beverly, professor in the Colleges of Nursing, Medicine, and Public Health at the University of Arkansas for Medical Sciences. Members of this population will be in their own homes and in nursing homes, hospitals, and assisted living facilities. Nurses must take a leadership role in caring for this population, Beverly emphasized.

Today the nursing workforce is inadequately prepared for the challenges of an aging population, Beverly said. Reimbursements outside acute care settings are not competitive; there is poor coordination among care settings; and there has been a lack of leadership and gerontological content throughout the nursing curriculum, from the associate to the bachelor's to the post-baccalaureate degree levels (Berman et al., 2005; IOM, 2008; Kovner et al., 2002).

Nurses also have been reluctant to take positions as decision makers within the health care system. As a result, chronic care tends to be relatively unmanaged, and there is a lack of emphasis on prevention and health promotion. In addition, Beverly said, practice constraints continue to be a problem throughout the health care system (Hooker et al., 2005; IOM, 2008).

Implementation and use of existing and new technology have been slow. Beverly highlighted a number of challenges related to the availability and use of technology: many nursing homes have either no or only one computer, which is usually reserved for billing purposes; there is little funding for either equipment or interventions using technology; very little money is available to place electronics into nursing homes to enable early interventions; and electronic health records have not been adopted widely in geriatric care practices (Committees on Energy and Commerce, Ways and Means, and Science and Technology, 2009; Hillestead et al., 2005).

Despite the abundance of challenges, Beverly cited accomplishments in long-term care and geriatric nursing led and supported by the John A. Hartford Foundation, the Geriatric Nurse Leadership Academy, the Donald W. Reynolds Foundation, stateside education consortia in Oregon and Minnesota, and the Sigma Theta Tau International Center for Nursing Excellence in Long-Term Care. For example, Sigma Theta Tau's Geriatric Nurse Leadership Academy just produced its first cohort of 16 nurses. The program "has had phenomenal results," said Beverly, "and we will be moving into our second year this spring."

Beverly offered three recommendations to the committee. First, a well-prepared long-term care workforce is essential for providing quality health care for older adults. There needs to be a strong pipeline, starting in middle schools and high schools, that leads to registered nurse programs. Also, the in-home health care curriculum is neither mandatory nor standardized in nursing education currently. "Nursing needs to play a role in making sure we have a strong curriculum that includes topics such as dementia and other topics." In particular, Beverly said that geriatric curricula in all registered nurse programs need to be reviewed "because a lot of programs say, 'we don't have a stand-alone [unit] but we integrate it,' but then when you look for where it is integrated, it's not." All registered nurses working in assisted living facilities, in nursing homes, or in home health care need to have adequate preparation in geriatric nursing. Closer relationships are also needed with geriatric nursing centers, which are supported through a federally funded program to provide education for health care professionals, noted Beverly.

Second, Beverly suggested that nurses must participate in and influence any major health care discussions about long-term care. Nurses "have not been aggressive in positioning ourselves to be part of that decision making," she said. Evidence-based models of care need to be incorporated into the health care delivery system, with the most appropriate provider paired with the right need. The role of registered nurses should be clearly articulated in every aspect of long-term care, and reimbursement systems should be rebalanced to embrace the full use of registered nurses.

Third, Beverly suggested a greatly increased use of technology. It should be applied in homes, in nursing homes, and in assisted living facilities. It should be used to improve education in schools and the delivery of nursing care. Also, in the form of electronic health records, the use of technology can greatly improve the coordination of care.

EVERCARE MODELS OF NURSING

Chronic diseases account for 75 percent of the nation's health care spending, and about two-thirds of the rise in health care spending is due to the increase in the prevalence of treatable chronic diseases, said Lynda Hedstrom, senior director of clinical services for Ovations. Yet vulnerable elders—people 65 and older who are at moderate or high risk for functional decline or death in the next 2 years—receive only about half of the recommended care (Wenger et al., 2003). "The idea that 100 people turn 60 every 13 minutes either keeps you up at night with anxiety or gives you some excitement about possibilities for the future," said Hedstrom.

The Evercare model that was developed by Ovations is based on special needs plans (sometimes known as SNPs) created by the Medicare Modernization Act of 2003. The special needs plans constitute a category of Medicare advantage plans that are designed to attract and enroll Medicare beneficiaries who fall into certain special needs demographics, including people who are institutionalized, who are eligible for both Medicare and Medicaid, or who have severe or disabling conditions. Hedstrom said that the plans go beyond the minimum that Medicare offers to provide care that is unique or special to their populations, such as transportation benefits or preventive dentistry for community-based members of the plan.

The Evercare model focuses on developing personalized health care plans, preventive services, and support for caregivers. It is designed to improve the coordination of care, enhance the quality of care by treating recipients at home, control costs, and produce outcomes important to these populations. With leadership from nurses, nurse practitioners, and care managers, the program monitors health status, manages chronic diseases, facilitates communication, avoids inappropriate hospitalizations, helps beneficiaries move from high risk to lower risk on the care continuum, aligns advance care planning with patient goals, and offers palliative care services.

Hedstrom described several studies that have demonstrated the benefits of this approach to care. In nursing homes, it reduces hospitalization (Kane et al., 2004), improves the cost effectiveness of care (Kane et al., 2003), and enhances family satisfaction (Kane et al., 2002). "Our family satisfaction surveys are still above 97 percent for that model," said Hedstrom.

In the community setting, the Assessing Care of Vulnerable Elders (ACOVE) project undertaken by RAND Health demonstrated improved geriatric care. The study developed quality indicators for medical conditions (e.g., chronic obstructive pulmonary disease, heart failure, diabetes, depression) and geriatric conditions (e.g., dementia, delirium, mobility disorders, incontinence) and found that Evercare providers did better than others in meeting these quality measures. The bottom line, said Hedstrom, is that the outcomes demonstrate "a significant improvement by our nursing interventions."[1]

Hedstrom drew several conclusions from these study results; she noted that care provided by physicians is generally good for medical conditions. However, when physicians partner with nurses in the Evercare model to provide care, there is significant improvement in quality indicators for geriatric conditions. According to clinical measures, patients without Evercare nurse contact receive worse care.[2] Hedstrom noted that nurses directly impact the quality and cost of health care.

These observations raise several intriguing questions, observed Hedstrom. Is the U.S. health care system ready to accept nurses as full partners in the provision of care, even to the extent of having independent and competitive practices? Would the health care system be willing to pay nurses directly? And what would have to change in terms of education, policy, and reimbursement practices for this to happen?

RESPONSES TO QUESTIONS

In response to a question about increasing the diversity of the nursing workforce to care for the aging population, Beverly noted that Hispanics and African Americans are underrepresented in the nursing profession.

---

[1] Wenger, N. 2009. Director, Assessing Care of Vulnerable Elders, RAND Corporation. Personal communication to David C. Martin, National Medical Director, Clinical and Quality Innovations, Ovations, October 29.

[2] Ibid.

However, many direct care workers are African Americans, often working near their own communities and demonstrating a love for caring for older adults. Not all of these individuals want to go into nursing, because they are very happy with what they are doing, "but there is a percentage—roughly expected to be around 30 percent—who would want to move into nursing, and I think it is up to us to try to move [them] on," said Beverly. For example, at an aging center in West Memphis, Arkansas, an African-American geriatrician and education director who is a nurse have been recruiting in churches, schools, and wherever they can show potential students that "there is a place for me there."

Another questioner asked about foreign-trained nurses in long-term care settings; Beverly observed that the content of their education is uncertain, although in the United States "we have not been consistently educating nurses at all levels to have expertise or at least a baseline in geriatric nursing and leadership." Beverly noted that most registered nurses (RNs) who work in nursing homes operate in director-of-nursing positions. If all nursing homes and other long-term care facilities had computers and access to the Internet, online assessments and training for geriatric care could be delivered to all nurses in those settings, regardless of their educational background and roles within the long-term care facilities.

Hedstrom added that it is important to demonstrate the value of nurses and nursing interventions in long-term care settings. Such information could help make it possible to reimburse nurses, especially advanced practice nurses, for the contributions they make to better health care. For example, the studies done by Ovations of the Evercare model originated from a desire to know how to spend limited funds most effectively, but they also demonstrated in a public way the value of nursing.

In response to a question about the stigma that sometimes surrounds long-term care and the possibility of moving such care into the community, Hedstrom replied that "we ought to have neighborhood nurses, church nurses, synagogue nurses—I think that nurses bring a level of care to their communities wherever they are." If nursing were more visible in these settings, people would be more willing to pay for the value nurses add. "The more we can define and make visible the special effects of nurses, the better," said Hedstrom.

Beverly observed that the visibility of nurses is increasing—they are becoming "more articulate, more open, and a champion for students' being in long-term care." She also pointed out that nurses could offer a valuable service by visiting with people who are caring for elderly family members and preparing assessments and plans for future care. "I don't know why every school of nursing does not have a house calls program, because it has a revenue stream and we, as nurses, have to become more understanding about developing businesses," said Beverly.

6

Testimony

Prior to the forum in Philadelphia, a variety of stakeholders and the public were invited to submit written testimony to the committee in four areas relevant to nursing care in the community: public health, community care, primary care, and long-term care. Those submitting written testimony were asked to describe innovative models in these four areas; barriers that nurses face in delivering care in the community; and how nurses could be further involved in advancing these areas of nursing across community settings.

Fifteen individuals at the forum provided prepared, oral testimony for the Initiative on the Future of Nursing; in most cases, these individuals or the organizations they represented also presented written testimony. Many important ideas and suggestions for the initiative emerged from this testimony and are summarized below. A number of other individuals attending the forum offered ad hoc observations and opinions on what was discussed. These comments are summarized at the end of this chapter. Like the presentations of the speakers, the testimony, observations, and opinions in this chapter should not be interpreted as positions or recommendations of the committee, the Robert Wood Johnson Foundation, or the Institute of Medicine.

Dana Egreczky, Vice President of Workforce Development
New Jersey Chamber of Commerce

For the past decade, the cost of health care has been among the top three concerns of business leaders, along with increasing taxes and fees and the lack of a qualified workforce, said Dana Egreczky, vice president of workforce development for the New Jersey Chamber of Commerce. Her state in particular has some of the highest health care costs in the country, which is why the New Jersey Chamber of Commerce made health care one of six planks in its Platform for Progress, a strategic initiative designed to give the state a more vibrant environment in which business can thrive. A partnership between the Robert Wood Johnson Foundation and the New Jersey Chamber of Commerce Foundation led to the New Jersey Nursing Initiative (NJNI), which is working to ensure that New Jersey has the well-prepared, diverse nursing workforce it needs to meet the demand for nursing in the twenty-first century. The grant has supported several new and innovative projects through the NJNI, such as an online service to help prospective students interested in nursing apply to multiple institutions around the state using a single application, an online service to optimize the number of clinical placements for nursing students, and development of a remediation language center for students.

Egreczky said the nursing community needs to reach out to the business community to ensure that nurses are available to improve the quality of life for patients and communities. Engaging the employer community has several benefits; Egreczky described three of these benefits. First, business leaders can help elevate the discussion of the future of nursing from a health care argument to an economic development argument; for example, they can point out to policy makers that they will have to fire or not hire new people as health care costs increase. "And if we have learned anything in the last few months, under the current economic crisis, it is that nothing puts as much fear into a politician's heart as the loss of jobs among the electorate. So use that to your advantage," said Egreczky.

Second, the business community can advocate for nurses' vision of the future. Nurses can use the high costs of health care—in terms of direct costs, lost productivity, and days away from work—to engage the interests of business leaders. Business leaders need to know that the looming crisis being generated by these costs is both "foreseeable and avoidable." However, they will not get involved unless the nursing community is unified. Egreczky also cautioned against asking the business community to support actions that would raise taxes or fees and she suggested approaching small, young companies as well as large, established companies in building support for nursing. Egreczky said, "When you seek a spokesperson, consider recruiting the president of a small company that is truly representative of the world of business and therefore truly feeling the pain of increasing percentages of revenue that employee health care costs are absorbing."

Finally, "never underestimate the power of a third-party broker that can exert pressure on the system," Egreczky said. The business community can make the case that rising health care costs will cause fewer people to have jobs, which will degrade the regional tax basis. "That is enough to make elected officials, college professors, and regulatory mavens—the very people we need to influence—sit up and take notice."

Skip Voluntad, Volunteer
AARP

Nurses are a vital link between patients and safe, high-quality health care, said Pioquinto (Skip) Voluntad, a volunteer with AARP. Though their role is often taken for granted, nurses are "touch points in nearly every interaction between the patient and the provision of care." AARP works with policy leaders, states, and the nursing community to increase awareness of the role that nurses play and the dire situation that the health care system must face unless the supply of highly skilled nurses is increased.

Voluntad described himself as a 79-year-old diabetic male with kidney failure. "I work with the primary care doctor and a kidney specialist, and I would not be here today to offer this testimony were it not for their knowledge and abilities. But I needed more. It was my great fortune that the nurses who work with my doctors also offer a great wealth of knowledge, and they are readily available when I have questions or need refills on my prescriptions. Many of them made it a point to know me personally, by phone when I could not see them in person. They all know me as Skip."

Voluntad noted that visiting nurses have checked on his diabetic treatments, monitored his blood pressure, and helped with his medicine doses at home, saving both him and his doctor considerable time. They have helped him with his living will. In addition, Voluntad's son had several operations, and during the year before his death, nurses were a great comfort to him, to Voluntad, and to the rest of the family.

Because of his exposure to the health care system, Voluntad learned from nurses that they were puzzled as to why so few Asian Americans in the surrounding community took advantage of the health care offered by the Delaware County Memorial Hospital. He teamed up with other

Asian-American activists in the community and with nurses to better understand and remove barriers to care. One of the greatest barriers was a language barrier. "The solutions to this problem required no new technology, no complex information systems, no new funding formulas—just care, common sense, and commitment," said Voluntad. Nurses and other health care professionals created a neighborhood response team and arranged for translators. In addition, hospital departments offered classes to members of the Asian-American community. A program available to all community members in eight different languages greatly increased the comfort levels of Asian Americans visiting the hospital, contributing to a 20 percent increase in the number of patients from the Asian-American community.

"Why were they successful?" Voluntad asked. "Because trying to understand patients' needs—medical and otherwise—is what nurses do." At the same time, nurses learned about family relationships, dietary differences, and philosophical distinctions between Eastern and Western medicine. "Is this kind of effort enough to solve the enormous health care challenges that we face? Certainly not. But just as certainly without including nurses as a key part of the solution we cannot succeed, which is why AARP supports an increased focus on advanced nursing education to ensure that we all have highly skilled nurses when and where we need them," concluded Voluntad.

Samuel Albrecht, Executive Director
Commission for Case Manager Certification

Case management and care coordination are well-established practices primarily performed by registered nurses, said Samuel Albrecht, executive director of the Commission for Case Manager Certification (CCMC). Certified case managers work collaboratively across the entire spectrum of the health and human services continuum to assess, plan, implement, coordinate, monitor, and evaluate the options and services required to meet their clients' needs. Certification, which requires specialized skills and knowledge, is based on field research and a test.

Nurse case managers work in a variety of settings, but they perform care coordination and case management in community health to a greater extent than in any other arena, said Albrecht. In community health settings, nurse case managers use appropriate medical, psychosocial, and community resources to meet patient's holistic needs for high-quality and timely access to necessary services. Nurse case managers also lead and participate in multidisciplinary teams to achieve desired outcomes using evidence-based guidelines.

Many models being considered as part of health care reform contain a care coordination component. As new models of health care are piloted and improved, care coordination and case management will remain essential elements, said Albrecht. In the future, nurse case managers will increase their use of technology—including electronic medical records, data mining, and biometric data—to obtain information and communicate with patients, providers, and other stakeholders. Through continued certification, nurse case managers will continue to seek optimal outcomes for their clients and ultimately for the public.

Gloria McNeal, Professor of Nursing and Associate Dean for Community and Clinical Affairs, University of Medicine and Dentistry of New Jersey School of Nursing

Gloria McNeal, serves as a project director for a nurse-managed mobile health care clinic, in addition to her roles at the University of Medicine and Dentistry of New Jersey School of Nursing. The clinic provides primary care services at 20 different locations in four cities in New Jersey. Its goal is to provide primary care services through advanced practice nurses in an interdisciplinary setting to patients who are uninsured. The services provided by the mobile clinic include diagnosis, management, and treatment for a variety of ambulatory care sensitive conditions. Due to grants totaling $3.5 million, the services provided by the mobile clinic are completely free to the clients it serves.

Several weeks ago, a client with four children came aboard the clinic's vehicle and said that even though she was covered by Medicaid, her physician had told her that he does not see more than 10 percent of his patients through Medicaid and that therefore he would not accept Medicaid coverage for her or her children. "That caused a light bulb to go off in my head," said McNeal. "Just because you are insured does not guarantee access." As a result, the clinic has begun providing services to both uninsured and underinsured patients. McNeal has approached third-party payers to explain the role of the mobile nurse-managed clinic and to ask if they would reimburse the clinic's care. However, the payers responded that because the clinic is mobile and not a fixed site, it technically does not exist and cannot be covered, despite the fact that the services are available around the clock and each call it receives is answered either in person or through an answering service. "My plea is to identify solutions and recommendations that will allow third-party payers to recognize mobile nurse-managed clinics, because it has been documented that they get into the communities and provide needed care," said McNeal.

Elaine Tagliareni, Professor and Independence Foundation Chair
Community College of Philadelphia

Over the past decade the Community College of Philadelphia has partnered with Drexel University and Thomas Jefferson University to participate in a Bridges to the Baccalaureate Program funded by the National Institutes of Health (NIH) to support minority students who are completing an associate degree. In addition, the program has obtained funding from a foundation to support 36 graduates of the program through their bachelor's degree, with most of the students engaging in community health activities in nurse-managed health clinics.

The results of the program have been "stunning," according to Elaine Tagliareni, professor and Independence Foundation chair at the Community College of Philadelphia. Ninety percent of the students have completed their bachelor's degree, and as of 2008, 60 percent had completed their master's degree, with an additional 17 percent currently enrolled in graduate programs. National statistics vary, but typically show that just over 20 percent of associate degree recipients and nurses prepared initially in baccalaureate programs continue their education, moving on to higher degree levels (HRSA, 2004a).

Even more spectacular, said Tagliareni, is that 100 percent of the graduates have returned to work with vulnerable populations in community-based settings. "Their work as advanced practice nurses has made a vital contribution to addressing health disparities and managing chronic care in the local community," noted Tagliareni.

This is a relatively small example, Tagliareni said, "but it packs a powerful message." Through faculty support, funding at the point of entry into nursing, and subsequent collaborative relationships throughout all levels of nursing, students from minority backgrounds can gain a new vision of what they can do and return to local communities as advanced practice nurses ready to give culturally sensitive care to vulnerable populations. Bringing programs such as this to scale in a reformed health care system will be vital to reducing health disparities and increasing the numbers of minority nurses, concluded Tagliareni.

Martha Dewey Bergren, Director of Research
National Association of School Nurses

School nurses represent a tremendous economic investment in the nation's children, said Martha Dewey Bergren, director of research at the National Association of School Nurses. The nation's 66,000 registered nurses who work in school settings straddle the boundaries between community, education, and home. They do not go into the community; they are already embedded in the community. They promote health, prevent injury and illness, provide 40 percent of child mental health services in the United States, and connect families and children to health insurance and a medical home. School nurses provide the only access to health care for many children who are homeless, immigrants, refugees, and underserved in both rural and urban areas. They are onsite champions for healthy eating, physical activity, indoor air quality, and green cleaning. They provide case management for children with asthma, diabetes, and anaphylactic food allergies. They also are integral to public health through their work in immunizations, disease surveillance, and dental, vision, and hearing screening.

However, one-quarter of the nation's children do not have a school nurse, Bergren said. On average, each school nurse serves 1,151 students and 2.2 schools. There is not a shortage of school nurses per se, but there is a shortage of positions for school nurses. In fact, surveys show that school nurses are the most satisfied of all nursing subspecialties, said Bergen.

To maximize the investment in school nurses, they need to have access to electronic health records. Already, more than half of school nurses are using such records, which helps them link students with primary care providers and community services. School nurses also have been engaged in some promising pilot projects in telehealth.

Today, school health is funded by the education system, which represents a cost shift from the health care system to the education system. Instead, school health services should be funded from outside the education system, Bergren said.

Sharon Moffatt, Chief of Health Promotion and Disease Prevention
Association of State and Territorial Health Officials

Public health nursing is a critical component of public health and the nation's health system, said Sharon Moffatt, chief of health promotion and disease prevention for the Association of State and Territorial Health Officials. Public health nurses have historically comprised 20 percent of the public health workforce at the state and local levels. They provide maternal-child health, respond to disasters ranging from floods to terrorism to hurricanes, offer a unique population-based knowledge, serve as a link between direct care and population-based practice, contribute to health policy, and have a long history of adapting to the changing health needs of communities.

In Vermont, for example, Moffat said that public health nurses are members of community health teams that work with primary care offices to connect high-risk patients to community resources. The public health nurse brings to the team expert knowledge of population-based analysis, state and local resources, and evidence-based interventions. They can identify gaps in services and barriers to access and can foster change at the community and state levels. Community health teams in Vermont are funded by private insurers, Medicaid, and state general funds, and in the very near future teams also will be funded by Medicare.

Public health nurses have an opportunity to make a significant contribution to a more accessible, affordable, and accountable health care system. Yet states are experiencing serious declines in public health nursing positions, Moffatt said. A prominent role for public health nurses in community health teams would be an excellent way to link clinical health care with public health and should be considered by the committee as it develops its recommendations.

Teresa Garrett, Chief Public Health Nursing Officer
and Deputy Director, Utah Department of Health

One Wednesday shortly before the forum, Teresa Garrett, the chief public health nursing officer and deputy director at the Utah Department of Health, spent 8 hours in her car, 6 hours at an H1N1 mass vaccination clinic, 2 hours on e-mail, and 1 hour on a conference call while she was driving. She dealt with three telephone calls from reporters and two calls from concerned legislators about the new mammogram guidelines. She walked 1,623 steps, drank four bottles of water, ate at McDonald's, and took a nap at a rest stop for 20 minutes. Garrett said that her situation is not much different from those of her colleagues in public health nursing. "Our jobs are hard, challenging, and the experience of a lifetime."

Garrett's greatest concern is the public health nursing shortage. In 1980, public health nurses represented 39 percent of the public health workforce. Today they are somewhere between 11 and 15 percent of that workforce, said Garrett. In a recent study, 30 of 37 states surveyed reported that the loss of public health nurses is their greatest concern in the deterioration of the public health system (Perlino, 2006). Public health nurses are the critical link in changing behaviors and improving the health of entire populations. They promote health, disease prevention, and social change and have a unique ability to reach across cultural divides. "These are the things that we will need in a truly reformed health system," Garrett said.

A variety of factors are contributing to the current public health nursing shortage, including the aging population of nurses, poorly funded public health systems, limited advocacy for public health, a growing shortage of faculty who understand how to teach public health nursing, curricula that do not adequately cover public health or community nursing, and the overall invisibility of public health nurses. To counter these trends, Garrett said that public health nurse leadership development needs to be nurtured, resources are required to rebuild the public health nursing infrastructure, and a new infrastructure is needed to provide interventions to vulnerable and at-risk populations that represent the weakest link in the health care system.

Tina Johnson, Director of Professional Practice & Health Policy
American College of Nurse-Midwives

The Maryland General Women's Health Associates serves one of the most at-risk communities in the city of Baltimore, said Tina Johnson, director of professional practice and health policy for the American College of Nurse-Midwives, who serves as a certified nurse midwife for the group. Yet this obstetric service has the lowest cesarcan section rate in all of Maryland, with "decreased morbidity and mortality and decreased costs to the health care system," said Johnson.

For many clients of the service, nurse midwives are the only health care providers they have encountered since childhood. They enter the service in desperate need of nutritional and exercise counseling, relationship and parenting skills, immunizations, dental care, mental health care, social services, smoking cessation, addiction services, and a wealth of other services, Johnson said. The women are encouraged to use the midwives' 24-hour telephone triage system, which builds trust, enhances communication, and decreases emergency room visits and hospital stays. As women progress throughout pregnancy, labor, delivery, and the postpartum period, midwives are there "all along the way," said Johnson, "diagnosing and treating their chronic and acute conditions, their asthma, bronchitis, skin rashes, and any infections that crop up, and managing their diabetes, preeclampsia, and many other health care needs." If the women are able to continue with their care through the program, it can be continuous throughout their lifespan, though most are covered only during pregnancy.

The nurse midwives at Maryland General also provide education and training for family practice residents at the University of Maryland. The residents work one on one with midwives in the labor and delivery unit, learning firsthand how to assess, evaluate, appropriately treat, and communicate with clients. "The collaborative care model in place at this institution requires a high degree of trust and respect among providers, with each team member providing care, perspective, and expertise. This philosophy is modeled for the residents, resulting in a broader knowledge base and an enhanced interdisciplinary educational experience," said Johnson.

Given the many advantages of this program, why aren't more communities using collaborative midwife models for obstetric and primary care for women? Unfortunately, there are many barriers, Johnson said. The Maryland General Women's Health Associates cannot readily collect the data needed to demonstrate adequately the effectiveness of its interventions because patients are admitted to the hospital under the name of the attending physician, not the name of the midwife. The group has not been able to convince the hospital administration to grant admitting privileges for certified nurse midwives, nor can they practice to the full scope of their licensure. For example, in the State of Maryland and many others, certified nurse midwives must have a signed collaborative agreement on file with the Board of Nursing to get a license. "This means essentially that you have to have a job before you can practice. You can't get a license until you already have a job, and people have difficulty starting practices or expanding services because of this." Additionally, midwives and other advanced practice nurses cannot be equitably reimbursed for all services in all settings by Medicare and Medicaid and other payers. Nor can they be paid for their services training residents or even their own midwifery students, because the slots available for midwifery and other nursing students are taken up by medical residents for whom the institution is paid, said Johnson.

"It is imperative that barriers to collaborative community care models such as these across the country be removed once and for all so that improved access to high-value primary care is available to everyone," Johnson concluded.

Susan Apold, President
New York State Association of Nurse Practitioners

"The nation's nurse practitioners stand ready to participate in the solution to the looming primary care crisis," said Susan Apold, president of the New York State Association of Nurse Practitioners. A century ago, fewer than 10 percent of physicians held a bachelor's degree, and the number one cause of death was infection. At that time the nation took a look at health care and made a conscious decision to change how it was done. A similar change is needed today, said Apold. The diagnosis and cure system that characterizes U.S. health care has become outdated. What is needed today is a prevention and management method of care. "There is more than enough work to go around for every health care provider in this nation, if we model the health care system the way it needs to be modeled," said Apold.

For nurse practitioners to be part of the solution, barriers to practice must be eliminated. Apold said that when she gets on a plane in New York and flies to New Mexico, "I no longer need any regulation to practice—it is an amazing phenomenon." The future of primary care depends on the full integration of all health care professionals practicing at the full scope of their licenses. Apold said that the regulation by states of nurse practitioners is not based on evidence or on best practices in primary care. In addition, the education of nurses and equitable reimbursements need to be re-examined. "We cannot continue to throw money at a system that does not work. We must pay for performance," concluded Apold.

Pat Ford-Roegner, Chief Executive Officer
American Academy of Nursing

Evidence-based, nurse-led interventions can improve the health and psychological resilience of individuals, families, and communities, said Pat Ford-Roegner, CEO of the American Academy of Nursing (AAN). Three years ago the AAN helped initiate the Raise the Voice campaign to end the invisibility of nursing. One of the first actions by that campaign was to call for the full integration of mental health services into the health care delivery system. In particular, older Americans with co-existing depression, anxiety disorder, or dementia need appropriate nursing care across all settings. "It is nurses who care for elders in long-term care, primary care, acute care settings, and the home." Ford-Roegner said that all nurses must have the capacity and competence to handle the full range of needs of older adults.

The AAN's Geriatric Nursing Collaborative is developing and disseminating core educational enhancements, curricula, and online guides for all nurses and all nursing programs. These resources will help nurses to care for and be able to recognize at least the basic mental health needs of the aging population, but this effort needs more funding and support to succeed across all practice and educational settings. For advanced practice nurses who specialize in psychiatric nursing, barriers to practice must be removed, particularly in regard to prescription of medication. In addition, much more needs to be done to work closer with mental health consumer organizations to reduce all barriers to the full integration of mental health and substance abuse services into primary care, concluded Ford-Roegner.

Andrew Rosenzweig, Assistant Clinical Professor
Brown University Medical School
and Medical Director, MedOptions

Some of the most challenging patients in long-term care are those with dementia, mental health disorders, and other behavioral health problems, said Andrew Rosenzweig, assistant clinical professor at Brown University Medical School and medical director for MedOptions. These patients can contribute to high levels of staff turnover and can even be responsible for workplace violence, which occurs more frequently in nursing homes than in any other workplace setting.

MedOptions, which is the largest provider of behavioral health care services to long-term care facility residents in four states, uses nurse-led multidisciplinary teams of psychiatrists, psychologists, social workers, physician assistants, and others to deliver care. A focus of the effort is to educate and empower the nursing staff in the facilities, "who are paramount to improving the quality of care of our patients and quality of life," said Rosenzweig. This approach has been able to overcome many of the challenges of long-term care, including workplace stress, dissatisfaction, and overreliance on medications for management of behavioral problems. "Our clinical model is based on what actually works, as opposed to what is easy to implement. We use behavioral management approaches and not just purely pharmacological approaches. And we involve staff and family members in the treatment team. We don't just focus on the resident. Instead [we] develop solid relationships with facility staff based on trust, availability, and creative problem-solving skills," said Rosenzweig.

The results of this approach have included reductions in hospital admissions, fewer emergency room visits, improved staff and family satisfaction, and improved compliance and survey results. "Positive outcomes occur naturally," Rosenzweig said.

David Smith, Research Professor
Drexel University School of Public Health

A recent article in *Health Affairs* titled "The Accumulated Challenges of Long-Term Care" (Smith and Feng, 2010) and a recent book titled *The Forensic Case Studies: Diagnosing and Treating the Pathologies of the American Health System* (Smith, 2009) both point out that the long-term care system now faces its most serious crisis of the past century, observed David Smith, research professor at the Drexel University School of Public Health's Center for Health and Quality. In the next four decades, there will be a fourfold increase in the number of people needing long-term care. Of more concern, there will be a dramatic shift from inpatient nursing home settings to home- and community-based services. Nurses will be in the "hot seat," said Smith, as this transition occurs. In particular, serious problems in terms of the quality of care can be expected to occur repeatedly in the long-term care system.

A way to ease this transition will be to move away from reliance on fee-for-service payments to models that have been pioneered in long-term care, such as the PACE (Program of All Inclusive Care for the Elderly) program and social health maintenance organizations, said Smith. In addition, the health care reform bill debated in Congress included provisions for people to purchase care in their own homes.

Debra Wolf, Associate Professor
Slippery Rock University

The use of information technologies can lead to greatly improved outcomes for the quality and safety of health care delivered to aging populations, said Debra Wolf, associate professor at Slippery Rock University. In one long-term care facility where the effects of innovative technology were documented, skin breakdowns in high-risk patients decreased by 75 percent, nursing turnover decreased by 74 percent, and nursing assistant turnover decreased by 40 percent, said Wolf.

The TIGER (Technology Informatics Guiding Education Reform) initiative depends on the need for nursing executives to envision and embrace accelerated adoption of technology using standards-based, interoperable technology that can support clinical decision making. Not only do such systems have the ability to stop drug-to-drug interactions or allergy-to-drug interactions, but they have the logic to alert nursing assistants to "not forget to turn Ms. Smith—she is at high risk. Don't forget to toilet Mr. Smith—he needs it every two hours," said Wolf.

Nurses need to design these systems, not information technology staff who do not understand nursing processes, said Wolf. The TIGER initiative also believes that education reform in nursing programs is needed to develop a workforce that is capable of using technology. This education, whether delivered through two-year or four-year programs, needs to teach prospective nurses how to look at workplace logic, how to question it, and how to design it. "This is redefining what meaningful use really is," said Wolf. "Nurses need to be actively involved at the national level with health information technology—advancing, guiding, and leading."

Gwen Foster, representing Juliet Santos
of the International Council for Corporate Health

The nation cannot afford today's spiraling health care costs, so prevention is essential, said Gwen Foster, who was representing Juliet Santos, president of the International Council for Corporate Health. Nurses must be trained to mentor and provide skills to people so that they undertake their own personal health reform, regardless of their inborn predispositions. "Faulty genes might load the gun, but it is lifestyle that pulls the trigger," said Foster. As an example, Foster cited a group of diabetics who were able to get their type 2 diabetes under control, despite a lack of health insurance and other resources. Nurse practitioners took the lead in home programs organized as health parties, where nurses in people's home gave them the skills and motivation to change.

Beyond prevention, nurses need to teach people to take personal responsibility for their health. Foster uses what she calls the FACES model—fun, accountable, credible, empowering, and sustainable. "We have to get out of the notion of blaming everybody else," she said. "We have to empower people and give them the skills so they can do it with us or without us."

Concluding Remarks

At the end of the forum, moderator Josef Reum invited members of the audience to comment on ideas they had heard during the event or to add points that they had not heard. This final open-microphone session yielded many interesting observations from the audience. Like the testimony summarized above, these comments should not be interpreted as positions or recommendations of the committee, the Robert Wood Johnson Foundation, or the Institute of Medicine. The section below includes a summary of the remarks that were offered by members of the audience at the forum:

- Public health nurses have important roles to play in advancing health policy no matter what the setting—in front of a school board, in their communities, in the state legislature, or at the federal level.
- Education programs will never be able to fully prepare future nurses for all the roles they must fill, which means that programs

for new nurses are essential, especially programs that connect novice nurses with experienced mentors in community settings, said one forum participant.

- Nursing needs to reflect the diversity of society, which will require that nurses from diverse populations assume leadership roles, said a member of the audience. These leaders could help recruit, retain, and promote the next generation of nurses. The audience member noted that there needs to be better communication between community health nurses and nurses in academia about the importance of nurses' roles in maintaining health, no matter the setting in which a nurse works.

- On a global scale, more than two-thirds of the world's population is not white. Issues of disparities, diversity, and inequities are prevalent in the United States, but the face of nursing in the United States does not reflect the global reality, said one forum participant. U.S. nursing should be seen in a global context, where the majority of nurses are nonwhite.

- Nurses need to be leaders in the shift of the health care system from an emphasis on diagnosis and treatment to an emphasis on wellness and prevention, suggested another member of the audience. With their specialized skills and perspectives, nurses are well positioned to help the health care system make this transition. Yet nursing education is today heavily focused on acute medical care, which requires changes in the curriculum to prepare nurses for a different kind of future.

- The health care system today is fragmented and based on payment models. One individual envisioned a project to build a continuous model of care that could start in 12 communities and could then lead the way to changes on a much broader scale. In such a model, nurses in different parts of the health care system, such as acute care nurses and public health nurses, would work together to ensure seamless transitions for health care recipients.

- U.S. nursing homes are in an emergency situation, said one forum participant. The majority of residents in these facilities are experiencing an absence of professional nursing care; there are not enough nurses employed in nursing homes, so the average resident receives just a half an hour a day of care from a registered nurse. The federal and state governments generally require limited coverage of nursing homes by registered nurses, and these nurses are paid significantly less than their colleagues in hospitals, which creates serious recruitment and retention challenges. The participant offered a number suggestions for the committee to consider, including the following:

- o The number of registered nurses in nursing homes should increase;
- o Nurses should be able to provide health assessments and care management to residents while ensuring safe supervision of the unlicensed staff, who provide the majority of care;
- o There should be adequate proportions of federal and state funding to pay for the care of residents in nursing homes, and funding should be targeted to nurse staffing and to adequate compensation for registered nurses; and
- o A national campaign should be launched to recruit future nurses into careers of caring for older adults.

- For nurses and other health care professionals to deliver the best possible care, they need access to information about evidence-based interventions, said a member of the audience. Nurses therefore need to be prepared to use information technologies to access the information that will drive health care in the future.
- Nurses need to be able to cross institutional boundaries to prevent the "siloing" that is so prevalent in health care. A nurse practitioner should be able to run a clinic in a school while also being the school nurse and proving opportunities for students with diverse backgrounds to become interested in nursing, said one forum participant.
- A profile of nursing needs to be done in different settings, looking at age, retirement plans, expertise, leadership, the potential for nurses to move from one setting to another, and so on, suggested one individual.
- A television show about nursing could demonstrate the full diversity of what nurses offer, particularly in creating collaboration across disciplines, said one participant. Similarly, the participant said that the President's cabinet should not be considered complete unless there is a nurse at the table.
- Nurses and other health care providers who want to work in the community need to put aside stigma and social distinctions and create a new model of training that deviates from the past emphasis on acute illness, said another member of the audience.

- Many physicians are frustrated because they lack the skills to be effective in the community, said one forum participant. Nurses could forge a partnership with physicians around the need for a common set of training experiences that will permit both groups of professions to meet the challenges of community-based medicine.
- Education models must foster creativity, empowerment, and leadership if nurses are to make the changes needed for better health of everyone in a community, concluded another participant.

A

References

AANP (American Academy of Nurse Practitioners). 2007. *Nurse practitioner cost-effectiveness.* Washington, DC: AANP.

Berman, A., M. Mezey, M. Kobayashi, T. Fulmer, J. Stanley, D. Thornlow, and P. Rosenfeld. 2005. Gerontological nursing content in baccalaureate nursing programs: Comparison of findings from 1997 and 2003. *Journal of Professional Nursing* 21(5):268-275.

Christensen, C. 1997. *The innovator's dilemma: When new technologies cause great firms to fail.* Cambridge, MA: Harvard Business School Press.

———. 2009. *Key concepts—Disruptive innovation.* http://www.clayton christensen.com/disruptive_innovation.html (accessed December 16, 2009).

Committees on Energy and Commerce, Ways and Means, and Science and Technology (Majority Staff). 2009. *Summary of Title IV—Health Information Technology for Economic and Clinical Health Act.* Washington, DC: U.S. House of Representatives.

Craven, G., and S. Ober. 2009. Massachusetts nurse practitioners step up as one solution to the primary care access problem: A political success story. *Policy, Politics, & Nursing Practice* 10(2):94-100.

Dilley, J. 2009. *Research review: School-based health interventions and academic achievement.* Olympia, WA: Washington State Department of Health, Washington State Office of Superintendent of Public Instruction, and Washington State Board of Health.

Hansen-Turton, T., L. Line, M. O'Connell, N. Rothman, and J. Lauby. 2004 (unpublished). *The nursing center model of health care for the underserved.* Submitted to the Centers for Medicare & Medicaid Services, June 2004. (Available from the National Nursing Centers

Fairman Consortium, 260 S. Broad Street, 18th Floor, Philadelphia, PA 19102.)

Hansen-Turton, T., A. Ritter, and R. Torgan. 2008. Insurers' contracting policies on nurse practitioners as primary care providers: Two years later. *Policy, Politics, & Nursing Practice* 9(4):241-248.

Hansen-Turton, T., A. Ritter, and B. Valdez. 2009. Developing alliances: How advanced practice nurses became part of the prescription for Pennsylvania. *Policy, Politics, & Nursing Practice* 10(1):7-15.

Hillestead, R., J. Bigelow, F. Girosi, R. Meili, R. Scoville, and R. Taylor. 2005. Can electronic record systems transform health care? Potential health benefits, savings, and costs. *Health Affairs* 24(5).

Hooker, R., D. Cipher, and E. Sekscenski. 2005. Patient satisfaction with physician assistant, nurse practitioner, and physician care: A national survey of Medicare beneficiaries. *Journal of Clinical Outcomes Management* 12(2):88-92.

HRSA (Health Resources and Services Administration). 2004a. *The registered nurse population: Findings from the National Sample Survey of Registered Nurses.* Rockville, MD: HRSA.

———. 2004b. *What is behind HRSA's projected supply, demand, and shortage of registered nurses.* Rockville, MD: HRSA.

IOM (Institute of Medicine). 1988. *The future of public health.* Washington, DC: National Academy Press.

———. 2002. *The future of the public's health in the 21st century.* Washington, DC: The National Academies Press.

———. 2008. *Retooling for an aging America: Building the health care workforce.* Washington, DC: The National Academies Press.

Jencks, S. F., M. V. Williams, and E. A. Coleman. 2009. Rehospitalizations among patients in the Medicare fee-for-service program. *New England Journal of Medicine* 360(14):1418-1428.

Kane, R. L., S. Flood, G. Keckhafer, B. Bershadsky, and Y. S. Lum. 2002. Nursing home residents covered by Medicare risk contracts: Early findings from the Evercare evaluation project. *Journal of the American Geriatrics Society* 50(4):719-727.

Kane, R. L., G. Keckhafer, S. Flood, B. Bershadsky, and M. S. Siadaty. 2003. The effect of Evercare on hospital use. *Journal of the American Geriatrics Society* 51(10):1427-1434.

Kane, R. L., S. Flood, B. Bershadsky, and G. Keckhafer. 2004. Effect of an innovative Medicare managed care program on the quality of care for nursing home residents. *Gerontologist* 44(1):95-103.

Karoly, L. A., P. W. Greenwood, S. S. Everingham, J. Hoube, M. R. Kilburn, C. P. Rydell, M. Sanders, and J. Chiesa. 1998. *Investing in our children: What we know and don't know about the costs and benefits of early childhood interventions.* Santa Monica, CA: RAND.

Kovner, C., M. Mezey, and C. Harrington. 2002. Who cares for older adults? Workforce implications of an aging society. *Health Affairs* 21(5):8-89.

Lee, P. V., and D. Lansky. 2008. Making space for disruption: Putting patients at the center of health care. *Health Affairs (Millwood)* 27(5):1345-1348.

Meadow, S. 2007. *Potentially preventable hospitalizations among Medicare home health patients* (poster presentation to the Agency for Healthcare Research and Quality). http://www.cms.hhs.gov/ResearchGenInfo/Downloads/CMSPosterPresentationAHRQ2007.pdf (accessed February 11, 2010).

Mehrotra, A., M. C. Wang, J. R. Lave, J. L. Adams, and E. A. McGlynn. 2008. Retail clinics, primary care physicians, and emergency departments: A comparison of patients' visits. *Health Affairs (Millwood)* 27(5):1272-1282.

Mehrotra, A., H. Liu, J. L. Adams, M. C. Wang, J. R. Lave, N. M. Thygeson, L. I. Solberg, and E. A. McGlynn. 2009. Comparing costs and quality of care at retail clinics with that of other medical settings for 3 common illnesses. *Annals of Internal Medicine* 151(5):321-328.

Olds, D. L., H. Kitzman, C. Hanks, R. Cole, E. Anson, K. Sidora-Arcoleo, D. W. Luckey, C. R. Henderson, Jr., J. Holmberg, R. A. Tutt, A. J. Stevenson, and J. Bondy. 2007. Effects of nurse home visiting on maternal and child functioning: Age-9 follow-up of a randomized trial. *Pediatrics* 120(4):e832-e845.

Perlino, C. 2006. *The public health workforce shortage: Left unchecked, will we be protected?* Washington, DC: American Public Health Association.

Rudavsky, R., C. E. Pollack, and A. Mehrotra. 2009. The geographic distribution, ownership, prices, and scope of practice at retail clinics. *Annals of Internal Medicine* 151(5):315-320.

Smith, D. 2009. *The forensic case files: Diagnosing and treating the pathologies of the American health system.* Hackensack, NJ: World Scientific.

Smith, D. B., and Z. Feng. 2010. The accumulated challenges of long-term care. *Health Affairs (Millwood)* 29(1):29-34.

Wenger, N. S., D. H. Solomon, C. P. Roth, C. H. MacLean, D. Saliba,
    C. J. Kamberg, L. Z. Rubenstein, R. T. Young, E. M. Sloss,
    R. Louie, J. Adams, J. T. Chang, P. J. Venus, J. F. Schnelle, and
    P. G. Shekelle. 2003. The quality of medical care provided to vulner-
    able community-dwelling older patients. *Annals of Internal Medicine*
    139(9):740-747.

B

Agenda

**Forum on the Future of Nursing:
Care in the Community**

Community College of Philadelphia
Great Hall (S2.19), Winnett Student Life Building
1700 Spring Garden, Philadelphia, PA 19130

December 3, 2009

AGENDA

12:30 pm	**Welcomes and Introductions** *Donna E. Shalala, University of Miami* *Stephen M. Curtis, Community College of Philadelphia* *Josef Reum, George Washington University*
12:45 pm	**Notes on Prescription for Pennsylvania** *Governor Edward Rendell*
	Committee Q&A and Discussion
1:30 pm	**Keynote Presentation** *Mary Selecky, Washington State Department of Health*

2:00 pm   **Panel on Community and Public Health**
                           Carol Raphael, Visiting Nurse Service of
                           *   New York*
                           Eileen Sullivan-Marx, University of
                           *   Pennsylvania School of Nursing*

                           Committee Q&A and Discussion

                           Presentation of Testimony

3:00 pm   **Break**

3:15 pm   **Panel on Primary Care**
                           Tine Hansen-Turton, National Nursing Centers
                           *   Consortium*
                           Sandra Haldane, Indian Health Service

                           Committee Q&A and Discussion

                           Presentation of Testimony

4:15 pm   **Panel on Chronic and Long-Term Services**
                           **   and Supports**
                           Claudia Beverly, University of Arkansas for
                           *   Medical Sciences School of Nursing*
                           Lynda Hedstrom, Ovations-Evercare by
                           *   UnitedHealthcare® Medicare Solutions*

                           Committee Q&A and Discussion

                           Presentation of Testimony

5:10 pm   **Open-Microphone Listening Session: Visions**
                           for the Future of Nursing

5:30 pm   **Closing Remarks**
                           Josef Reum, George Washington University

5:35 pm   **Forum Adjourn**

C

Speaker Biosketches

Claudia Beverly, Ph.D., R.N., FAAN, currently serves at the University of Arkansas for Medical Sciences (UAMS) campus as inaugural recipient of the Murphy Chair for Rural Aging Leadership and Policy in the College of Medicine; founding director of the Arkansas Hartford Center of Geriatric Nursing Excellence; founding director of the Arkansas Aging Initiative, Donald W. Reynolds Institute on Aging; and professor, Colleges of Nursing, Medicine, and Public Health. Dr. Beverly's areas of specialty and research interests include geriatrics and integrated community-based systems of health care and social service delivery. Her work in the community spans 35 years and includes establishing eight Centers on Aging, each with a primary care clinic employing an interdisciplinary geriatric team and an education component. Dr. Beverly's work in nursing home policy includes being one of the founding members of the Arkansas Coalition for Nursing Home Excellence, the state's leader in the national Advancing Excellence in America's Nursing Homes. She is the recipient of various awards including selected in the first cohort, Robert Wood Johnson Nurse Executive Fellowship, and the UAMS Faculty Service Award.

Sandra Haldane, B.S.N., M.S., R.N., received her B.S.N. from Baylor University in 1981 and her M.S. in nursing and health care administration in 2006 from University of Alaska Anchorage. She has worked clinically in obstetrics, labor and delivery, medicine-surgery, and intensive care. Her management and leadership experiences were with the Alaska Area Native Health Service and the Alaska Native Medical Center and currently with Indian Health Service (IHS) at its headquarters in Rockville, Maryland. Ms. Haldane assumed the position of the IHS director, Division of Nursing, and IHS chief nurse in October 2003. In this position, she provides national guidance on nursing practice, policy, advocacy, budget justification, and support for a variety of programs and grants in nursing and Indian health. She oversees the following programs: Public Health Nursing, Community Health Representatives, Women's Health, and Nursing Recruitment. Ms. Haldane is a member of the Tsimshean Tribe of Metlakatla, Alaska.

Tine Hansen-Turton, M.G.A., J.D., vice president at the Public Health Management Corporation (PHMC), has earned a reputation as an effective change agent, systems-thinker, social innovator, and policy advocate. She assists PHMC and its affiliates with business and programmatic strategy, development, coordination, and implementation, as well as with policy development and state and national advocacy. Ms. Hansen-Turton serves as CEO of the National Nursing Centers Consortium (NNCC), a nonprofit organization supporting the growth and development of more than 250 nurse-managed health clinics, serving more than 2.5 million vulnerable people across the country in urban, suburban, and rural locations. She is also co-founder and executive director of Convenient Care Association, a national trade association of more than 1,250 emerging private sector-based retail health clinics with the capacity to serve 17 million people. Ms. Hansen-Turton has been instrumental in positioning nurse practitioners as primary health care providers globally.

Lynda R. Hedstrom, M.S.N., certified nurse practitioner, senior director, Clinical Services for Ovations-Evercare by UnitedHealthcare® Medicare Solutions, joined Evercare in 2005 to direct the Evercare community program in Georgia and joined the Professional Practices Team in 2008. The Profession Practices Team recently became the Clinical Services and Training Team responsible for core processes for Model of Care delivery for our Special Needs plans and Medicare Advantage plans. Ms. Hedstrom's background includes home health care and home health care administration. She graduated from North Park University for her B.S.N. and from Brenau University for her master's and nurse practitioner degrees.

Carol Raphael, M.P.A., is president and CEO of the Visiting Nurse Service of New York, the largest nonprofit home health agency in the United States. Prior to joining the Visiting Nurse Service of New York (VNSNY), Ms. Raphael held positions as director of operations management at Mt. Sinai Medical Center and executive deputy commissioner of the Human Resources Administration in charge of the Medicaid and public assistance programs in New York City. Ms. Raphael was a member of the Medicare Payment Advisory Commission (MedPAC) and of the New York State Hospital Review and Planning Council. She chairs the New York eHealth Collaborative, a public-private partnership working to advance the adoption of health information technology in New York State. She is also on the Boards of Excellus/Lifetime Health Care Company and Pace University and is a member of numerous advisory boards including those of the Henry Schein Company, the Harvard School of Public Health Policy and Management Program, the Atlantic Philanthropies Geriatrics Practice Scholars, the New York University School of Nursing, the Markle Foundation's Connecting for Health, and the Jonas Center for Nursing Excellence. In addition, she has served on many health policy committees including the Institute of Medicine's (IOM's) Committee to Study the Workforce for Older Americans.

Edward G. Rendell, J.D., Pennsylvania's forty-fifth governor, began a second term of office on January 16, 2007, following a landslide reelection victory. As governor, Rendell serves as chief executive of the nation's sixth most-populous state and oversees a $28.3 billion budget. Governor Rendell's unprecedented strategic investments have energized Pennsylvania's economy, revitalized communities, improved education, protected the environment, and expanded access to health care for all children and affordable prescription drugs for older adults. He championed and signed into law Pennsylvania's first comprehensive measure to substantially reform the local tax system by providing urgently needed property tax relief to homeowners. In 2008-2009 taxpayers will save nearly $800 million in the first year of statewide property tax relief from gaming revenues. From 1992 through 1999, Governor Rendell served as the one hundred and twenty-first mayor of the City of Philadelphia. Before serving as mayor, Rendell was elected district attorney of the City of Philadelphia for two terms from 1978 through 1985. An Army veteran, the governor is a graduate of the University of Pennsylvania (B.A., 1965) and Villanova Law School (J.D., 1968).

Josef Reum, Ph.D., is the interim dean of the School of Public Health and Health Services at the George Washington (GW) University. Prior to joining the GW faculty in 1993, Dr. Reum was CEO of the American Health Quality Association, which represents organizations that provide evaluation and quality improvement services to health care purchasers and providers. His administrative skills were also essential to his tasks as deputy director of the Local Initiative Funding Partners Program, a Robert Wood Johnson Foundation national program designed to promote innovation in the design and delivery of health care services. Dr. Reum has held leadership positions in six states, including commissioner of the Department of Mental Health, Developmental Disabilities and Substance Abuse (Indiana); deputy commissioner of the Department of Mental Retardation (Massachusetts); and director of the Anchorage Department of Health and Social Services (Alaska).

Mary C. Selecky has been secretary of the Washington State Department of Health since March 1999, serving under Governor Chris Gregoire and former Governor Gary Locke. Prior to working for the state, Ms. Selecky served for 20 years as administrator of the Northeast Tri-County Health District in Colville, Washington. Throughout her career, Ms. Selecky has been a leader in developing local, state, and national public health policies that recognize the unique health care challenges facing both urban and rural communities. As secretary of health, Ms. Selecky has made tobacco prevention and control, patient safety, and emergency preparedness her top priorities. She is known for bringing people and organizations together to improve the public health system and the health of people in Washington. Ms. Selecky has served on numerous boards and commissions; she is a past president of the Association of State and Territorial Health Officials, receiving the 2009 President's Meritorious Service award and the 2004 McCormack Award for excellence in public health, and is a past president of the Washington State Association of Local Public Health Officials. A graduate of the University of Pennsylvania, she has been a Washington State resident for 35 years.

Donna E. Shalala, Ph.D., FAAN, is chair, Robert Wood Johnson Foundation Initiative on the Future of Nursing, at the Institute of Medicine. She is president of the University of Miami and professor of political science. President Shalala has more than 30 years of experience as an accomplished scholar, teacher, and administrator in government and universities. She has also held tenured professorships in political science at Columbia University, the City University of New York (CUNY), and the University of Wisconsin, Madison. She served as president of Hunter College of CUNY from 1980 to 1987 and as chancellor of the University of Wisconsin, Madison from 1987 to 1993. In 1993, President Clinton appointed her U.S. Secretary of Health and Human Services (HHS) where she served for 8 years, becoming the longest-serving HHS secretary in U.S. history. She received the Presidential Medal of Freedom, the nation's highest civilian award, in 2008. She is a member of the Institute of Medicine.

Eileen Sullivan-Marx, Ph.D., C.R.N.P., FAAN, R.N., is an active international and national consultant on nurse practitioner and geriatric practice issues, and she brings her international leadership reputation and skills to the forefront for University of Pennsylvania nursing students. With a strong background as a primary care nurse practitioner, she teaches the foundation course on assessment, health promotion, and critical thinking at the undergraduate level and lectures throughout the undergraduate and graduate courses on such topics as care of frail older adults in the local and global communities, models of care and payment policy, reimbursement for advanced practice nurses, and business and economic issues in health care delivery. Dr. Sullivan-Marx's research area focuses on outcomes of care for frail older adults and sustaining models of care using advanced practice nurses locally and globally. To date, she has investigated predictors and outcomes of advanced practice nursing care that inform U.S. health policy. Dr. Sullivan-Marx oversees the School of Nursing's practice and community mission through oversight of Living Independently for Elders (LIFE), Healthy in Philadelphia Initiative, Penn Nursing Consultation Service, and the Center for Professional Development. The LIFE program is a nurse-managed Program of All-Inclusive Care for the Elderly, serving more than 360 members 24 hours per day, 7 days a week, with comprehensive integrated health and social services for older adults in West Philadelphia who are eligible for nursing home care but are able to remain at home through this model program.